Practical Clinical Psychopharmacology

SECOND EDITION

Practical Clinical Psychopharmacology

SECOND EDITION

WILLIAM S. APPLETON, MD

Assistant Clinical Professor of Psychiatry
Harvard Medical School

JOHN M. DAVIS, MD

Director of Research
Illinois State Psychiatric Institute
Professor of Psychiatry
University of Chicago
School of Medicine
Lecturer
University of Illinois
School of Medicine

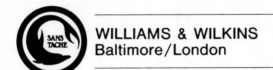

WILLIAMS & WILKINS
Baltimore/London

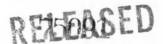

Copyright ©, 1980
The Williams & Wilkins Company
428 E. Preston Street
Baltimore, Md. 21202, U.S.A.

Made in the United States of America

Library of Congress Cataloging in Publication Date

Appleton, William S
    Practical clinical psychopharmacology.

    Bibliography: p.
    Includes index.
    1. Psychopharmacology. I. Davis, John M., 1933- joint author. II. Title. [DNLM:
1. Psychopharmacology. QV77 A652p]
RM315.A66 1979   616.8'918   78–24481
ISBN 0-683-00238-4

Composed and printed at the
Waverly Press, Inc.
Mt. Royal and Guilford Aves.
Baltimore, Md 21202. U.S.A.

To
*Jane, Amy, Lucy and Bill and
Judy, Richard and Kathy*

Foreword

This second edition on practical clinical psychopharmacology by William S. Appleton, M.D., and John M. Davis, M.D., succeeds once again in succinctly and completely explicating existing knowledge and recent advances in a rapidly expanding field. This volume, which includes essential topics organized in a convenient format, will have enormous benefit for both general practitioners and psychiatrists.

In the past quarter century, developments in psychopharmacology have led to dramatic changes in both the treatment and scientific investigation of psychiatric disorders. Therapeutic advances resulting from the development of new psychoactive drugs with proven efficacy in schizophrenia, mania, depression, anxiety and other clinical states have greatly changed psychiatric practice. These new treatments have differential effects that require careful matching of the patient's psychopathology with the specific treatment that is most likely to benefit the symptom picture and the clinical disorder. Experience with these new drugs, which have been shown to have varying neuropharmacologic modes of action, has demonstrated that they have different patterns of clinical efficacy. These findings support the concept that psychiatric disorders are discrete and heterogeneous.

In the research arena, the advent of psychoactive drugs has stimulated imaginative new hypotheses concerning CNS functioning in normal and abnormal states and has dramatically enhanced our understanding of the biochemical basis of mental illness. In clinical research, the need for therapeutic evaluation of drug efficacy and safety encouraged the development of controlled clinical trials and other improved research methods in clinical psychopharmacology.

Dr. Appleton and Dr. Davis have brought their respective talents to the writing of this volume. Dr. Appleton is an experienced clinician, skilled in psychotherapy as well as in pharmacotherapy, and an equally experienced teacher of psychopharmacology. Dr. Davis complements Dr. Appleton's clinical and teaching skills with his extensive knowledge of the literature and his skills in laboratory and clinical research, investigating the action of CNS drugs. Together, they have written a concise, comprehensive volume which translates complex research findings into a practical guide to assist clinicians in making basic decisions about the application of pharmacotherapy.

Gerald L. Klerman, M.D.

Gerald L. Klerman, M.D. is currently Administrator of the Alcohol, Drug Abuse, and Mental Health Administration in Rockville, Maryland. He is also Professor of Psychiatry (on leave) at the Harvard Medical School, Massachusetts General Hospital, where he was director of the Stanley Cobb Laboratories for Psychiatric Research. His main professional activities have involved research and teaching in clinical psychiatry and psychopharmacology, with an emphasis on depression and related affective disorders.

Among his honors is the Hofheimer Prize of the American Psychiatric Association, which was awarded in 1969 for his role as one of the Principal Investigators in the NIMH Collaborative Study of Phenothiazine Treatment of Acute Schizophrenia. In 1978, he shared the American Psychiatric Association Foundations' Fund Award in Research with his colleagues from the New Haven-Boston Collaborative Study on the Acute Treatment of Depression. Dr. Klerman is active in many professional societies and serves on the editorial boards of a number of professional journals. He was recently elected to a term at the Institute of Medicine.

Preface

In the seven years since the first edition much has been learned, but our original practical clinical purpose, desire for brevity, and reliance on scientific evidence rather than our own personal prescribing idiosyncrasies remains the same. We provide the practicing physician, psychiatrist and medical student with a guide through the confusing maze and vast literature of psychopharmacology. In a handful of revised summary tables we encapsulate the evidence of hundreds of well controlled studies. For those who wish further proof we have expanded the reference list without making it excessive.

All the latest drugs are included, along with new knowledge about the good and bad of the old ones and of the neurophysiology and neurochemistry of their action as well as of the illnesses they treat. Also, we have employed the new *Diagnostic and Statistical Manual* (DSM3) classification, one that has been largely influenced by the thinking of the field we attempt to summarize, psychopharmacology.

Much has been learned about the effectiveness of maintenance therapies in schizophrenia, mania and depression. Knowledge of lithium, the monoamine oxidase inhibitors and the drug treatment of agoraphobia has grown. The new techniques for precise measurement of the fate of these agents in patients has led to more rational amount and spacing of dosage. Thus, how much antidepressant to give or how often to administer a quick or slowly metabolized antianxiety or hypnotic agent can be determined.

The section on prevention and treatment of persistent (tardive) dyskinesia has been greatly expanded, and the description of the practical management of side effects re-written. Discussions of who should be medicated, for and with what, for how long, and with how much are included. A section on drug overdose appears once again.

A brand new table on "The Power of Psychoactive Drugs" summarizes the effectiveness of our major agents in the treatment and prevention of psychiatry's most significant conditions and compares our results to several significant drugs used in medicine and surgery. Happily, psychiatric medications work as well as those in other medical and surgical disciplines. Our advances in the last quarter century have been major and we can hold our heads up high.

William S. Appleton, M.D.
John M. Davis, M.D.

Contents

chapter ONE

Before Drug Therapy Begins

THE GENERAL DIAGNOSIS

To diagnose is to distinguish, to know, and to recognize a disease from its signs and symptoms. A diagnosis is the conclusion reached about the causes, natural course and/or treatment of disease.

Therapeutic action is taken based upon the diagnosis; it is not merely a labeling procedure. Ideally, diagnosis includes etiology, pathogenesis, stage of illness, differential response, prediction and prognosis.

Predicting the response to different treatments is implicit in the diagnostic process: i.e., knowing when the patient will do well on one treatment, but not on another. For example, consider a diagnosis of probable gram-positive infection versus infection with either gram-positive or gram-negative organisms. In the first case you would treat with agents effective against gram-positive organisms, but, in the latter, antibiotics effective against both gram-positive and gram-negative organisms are indicated.

Descriptive Syndrome Level

The etiologies and pathogenesis of psychiatric diseases are largely unknown. Now, because we must operate at the *descriptive syndrome level*, disagreement exists about both causation and therapeutic action. Nevertheless, psychiatrists generally agree that specific diseases do exist among psychiatric patients. Diagnostic classification enables a psychiatrist to predict course, prognosis and treatment responses.

Causation

Whatever causes psychosis, depression or neurotic disability,

1

psychological and pharmaceutical therapeutic treatments influence them all.

Therapeutic Action

Almost all psychiatrists agree that drug therapy is useful in treating schizophrenia, and most find drugs valuable in treating depression. However, there is much controversy about treating neurotics and patients with personality disorders with medication.

Diagnostic Process

Case Study

Make your diagnosis and prescribe therapy only after careful case study.

History

A careful personal and family history is necessary to help predict drug responses and possible side effects.

It has been claimed that there is an association between schizophrenia and social class. A methodological point is that social class is determined partly by such factors as education and occupation and, if a person has a severe disabling form of schizophrenia, there is a tendency for that person to drift downward in social class because they cannot attain distinction as reflected in educational and vocational criteria.

A number of studies indicate that there is a higher prevalence of schizophrenics of lower socioeconomic backgrounds and the distribution of the fathers of schizophrenics is the same as in the general population. This suggests that there is a "downward drift" of these individuals to the lower classes, rather than suggesting that aspects of the lower class cause schizophrenia.

Examination

Medical review is particularly critical if drug therapy is being considered. Psychological examinations are useful for evaluating intellectual abilities and some gross organic brain disorders. So are self-administered questionnaires and information from ward personnel, friends and family members. Psychological tests are useful as baseline data in organic and nonorganic disease for evaluating change.

Case Formulation

The above procedures should result in a case formulation, differential diagnosis and statement of unresolved issues requiring further investigation. Each diagnosis should include an explicit treatment plan and a review of the therapeutic modalities available.

THE DIAGNOSIS OF SCHIZOPHRENIA

What is schizophrenia? It is a persistent disturbance in perceiving or evaluating reality and it is of an unknown etiology. Similar symptoms produced by *known* causes are not considered schizophrenia:

- Toxic agents (infection, drug poison).
- Organic brain disease (senile disease, neoplasm).
- Sensory deficit (color blindness).
- Afferent abnormality (phantom limb).
- Extreme affects (elation, depression).
- Environmental agents (social, educational).

Transient perceptually disturbed states (e.g., sensory deprivation, hypnagogic states, intoxications and sleep deprivation) are also *not* included as schizophrenic disturbances.

Symptoms of Schizophrenia

Hallucinations

The patient experiences sensory perceptions without external stimuli.

The *auditory type* is most common, although schizophrenic hallucinations can occur in any sensory modality.

Hallucinations of sight, taste and odor may require an immediate search for an organic cause, since they are also present with organic illness.

Hallucinations also occur in toxic states, organic brain disease, malingerers, hysteria and epilepsy.

Delusions

Tenaciously held idiosyncratic false beliefs, that are not subject to change in evaluating new evidence or through persuasion are considered delusions. The patient uses these fabrications to explain his psychotic perceptual distortions and misevaluations.

Confused affective and cognitive state often exists prior to an acute schizophrenic episode. Delusions often occur as experiences of insight and illumination. What the patient previously "felt" or suspected, he now knows. As the doubt subsides, confusion and perplexity are relieved.

Delusions may also develop gradually as explanations for repeated rejections. The eccentric, inept preschizophrenic is unable to be realistically self-critical, and so develops delusions.

Delusions may be categorized as malevolent, benevolent or grandiose. They can be accompanied by fear (helplessness against the forces), anger (struggling against the forces), guilt (a justifiable punishment) or elation (self-misidentification, as God, for example.)

Beyond these symptoms are the seven Schneiderian first rank symptoms; (Corbett, 1978; Freedman et al., 1977):

- Hearing one's own thoughts.
- Voices conversing with one another about the patient.
- Voices keeping up a running commentary on the patient's behavior.
- Somatic hallucinations and passivity experiences.
- Thought insertion, withdrawal, or thought broadcasting.
- Feelings, impulses, or actions which are experienced as imposed on the person by outside agencies.
- Delusional perception.

And four Schneiderian second rank symptoms:

- Other hallucinations.
- Perplexity.
- Depressive and euphoric disorders of affect.
- Emotional blunting.

Thought Disorder

Bleuler, in 1950, was the first to consider thought disorder as the hallmark of schizophrenia. Most clinicians have focused on the quality of schizophrenic thought and have characterized thought disorder in various ways.

Goldstein was one of the first researchers to explore thought disorder in schizophrenic patients, and he characterized schizophrenic thinking as concrete: i.e., the inability to transcend immediate experience or the inability to adopt broader or general mental sets in which aspects of experience can be organized. Von Domarus characterized thought disorder as paralogical. According to Von Domarus, our logical processing establishes the reference of identity upon the basis of the identity of subjects: e.g., "Socrates is a man" and, "All men are mortal" leads to the logical conclusion that "Socrates is mortal." Paralogical processing establishes identity upon the basis of the identity of predicates: e.g., "Socrates is a man," and "I am a man" leads to the false conclusion that "I am Socrates." Werner felt that thought disorder was not paralogical but regressive, since such processing could be found in other cultures and in young children, whereas Arieti felt that thought disorder was paleological, in that it was a precursor of normal secondary process thought.

Most of the descriptive literature on thought disorder has distinguished it from normal thinking. Although many of the characteristics of thought disorder are not unique to schizophrenia, the accumulation of them is indicative of the illness. Yet, according to Johnston and Holzman (1979), there seem to be certain thought qualities which are associated with schizophrenia. These specific types of thought may not necessarily be evident in all schizophrenics, but their presence is often sufficient for serious consideration of a diagnosis of schizophrenia. The qualities that are found only in schizophrenics are contamination, incoherence and neologisms.

There are many other types of thought disorder; however, these symptoms can often be found within other psychiatric populations. For example, concreteness can occur in brain-damaged patients, while excessively fast or retarded thinking can be found respectively in mania and depression. Flight of ideas and tangential thinking can also be found in mania. Consequently, thought disorder is pathognomic only if organicity and affective illness can be ruled out. (See Table 1.1.).

In our laboratory we have shown that a precise psychological assessment of thought disorder, based on an item analysis of individual patients' responses, produces a score that is substantially abnormal in schizophrenic patients, and which becomes normalized following psychotropic drug treatment (Holzman and Hurt, unpublished). Furthermore, the time course of the improvement in the measurement of thought disorder exactly parallels the time course of improvement in symptom schizophrenia (Fig. 1.1).

Abnormal Emotion

Emotional blunting and flatness are typical in schizophrenia. Immediate differentiation from depressive apathy is difficult ex-

Table 1.1
Thought Disorder

Subtypes	Examples
Contamination	On the Rorschach from Card I, a patient stated: "A butterfly holding the world together because I see on both sides patterns of a map."
Incoherence	"I don't quite gather. I know one right and one left use both hands, but I can't follow the system that's working." (Mayer-Gross et al., 1969)
Neologisms	A patient reports that he was "accused of mitigation."
Illogical thinking	A patient gave her family IBM cards she punched in order to overcome communication difficulties.
Loosening of associations	"I'm tired. All people have eyes. Do you have glasses? I'm thirsty, can I have a glass of water?"
Poverty of content	"Well, er...not quite the same as, er...don't know quite how to say it. It isn't the same being in the hospital as er...working, er...the job isn't quite the same, er..." (Wing, 1971)
Condensation	(E) What does this saying mean: "One swallow doesn't make a summer." (S) "You can't enjoy everything in life just tasting the fruit one time."
Idiosyncratic word usage	"I have menu three times a day."
Clangs	On asking a patient the meaning of travesty, he reports, "I think of the treasure and the dynasty."
Concreteness	On asking a patient in what way are an orange and a banana alike, he reports that 'you peel them.''
Overinclusion	On asking the similarity between an orange and a banana, he reports, "They come from the earth."

cept through a history proving the latter to be temporary and phasic, and the former chronic.

Schizophrenics display inappropriate affect—a lack of harmony between thought and affect, which is often characterized as silliness. This finding in schizophrenia serves as an important diagnostic criterion.

Motor Signs

Motor abnormalities are not pathognomonic. They include grimacing, repetitive motor rituals, bizarre postures, mute states and inappropriate smiling. Catatonic postures are now rare.

General Symptoms Not Diagnostic of Schizophrenia

Panic, derealization, chaotic sexuality, depersonalization, pan-anxiety, impulsivity and pan-neurotic symptomatology do not, by themselves, allow a diagnosis of schizophrenia to be made (Table 1.2).

The present Diagnostic and Statistical Manual of the American Psychiatric Association gives detailed diagnostic criteria for mental illness and is in the process of revision from the Diagnostic and Statistical Manual Version II (DSM II) to the newer version (DSM III). As of this writing, DSM III has been accepted by the American Psychiatric Association, and for that reason we have specified in

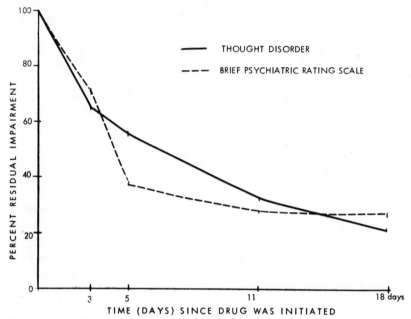

Figure 1.1. Symptom response to haloperidol (from Hurt et al., unpublished data).

Table 1.2

Common Categories of Schizophrenia-like Disorders

Schizophrenic Disorders	Paranoid Disorders	Psychotic Disorders (Not Elsewhere Classified)
Disorganized	Paranoia	Schizophreniform
Catatonic	Shared	Brief reactive psychosis
Paranoid	Acute	Schizoaffective
Undifferentiated	Atypical	Atypical psychosis (residual category)
Residual		

this book the latest draft of DSM III for the diagnosis of the schizophrenias and the affective disorders. It is possible that, after this book goes to press, the American Psychiatric Association may make further minor modifications in the DSM III; however the information included here is essentially an outline of the diagnostic criteria for schizophrenia and the affective disorders, which is correct at the present time.

Schizophrenic Disorders

Diagnostic Criteria

A. At least one symptom from among the following is present during a phase of the illness.
   (1) Bizarre delusions (patently absurd; has no basis in fact), such as delusions of being controlled, thought broadcasting, thought insertion, or thought withdrawal.
   (2) Somatic, grandiose, religious, nihilistic or other delusions without persecutory or jealous content.
   (3) Delusions with persecutory or jealous content, if accompanied by hallucinations.
   (4) Auditory hallucinations in which either a voice keeps up a running commentary on the individual's behaviors or thoughts or two or more voices converse with each other.
   (5) Auditory hallucinations with content having no apparent relation to depression or elation, and not limited to one or two words or occasions.
   (6) Incoherence, marked loosening of associations, markedly illogical thinking or marked poverty of content of speech, associated with at least one of the following:
      (a) Blunted, flat or inappropriate affect.
      (b) Delusions or hallucinations.
      (c) Catatonic or other grossly disorganized behavior.
B. Above symptoms in A impair two or more areas of daily function: e.g., work, social relationship, and self-care.
C. *Chronicity:* Signs of the illness have lasted continuously for at least 6 months at some time and the individual now has some signs of illness. The 6-month period must include an active phase during which there were symptoms from A with or without a prodromal or residual phase, as defined below.
   Prodromal Phase: A clear deterioration in functioning not due

to a primary disturbance of mood or to substance abuse, and involving at least *two* of the symptoms below.

Residual Phase: Following the active phase of the illness, at least *two* of the symptoms below, not due to a primary disturbance in mood or to substance abuse.

Prodromal or Residual Symptoms:

(1) Social isolation or withdrawal.

(2) Marked impairment in role functioning as wage-earner, student, homemaker.

(3) Markedly eccentric or peculiar behavior: e.g., collecting garbage, talking to self in corn field or subway, or hoarding food.

(4) Impairment in personal hygiene and grooming.

(5) Blunted, flat or inappropriate affect.

(6) Speech that is tangential, vague, overelaborate, circumstantial, or metaphorical.

(7) Bizarre ideation, or magical thinking: e.g., superstitiousness, clairvoyance, telepathy, "sixth sense," "others can feel my feelings," overvalued ideas, ideas of reference, or suspected delusions.

(8) Unusual perceptual experiences: e.g., recurrent illusions, suspected hallucinations.

    Examples: Six months of prodromal symptoms with 1 week of symptoms from A; no prodromal symptoms, with 6 months of symptoms from A; no prodromal symptoms with 2 weeks of symptoms from A and 6 months of residual symptoms; 6 months of symptoms from A, apparently followed by several years of complete remission, with 1 week of symptoms in A in current episode.

D. The full depressive or manic syndrome (Criteria A and B of Depressive or Manic Episode) is either *not* present, developed after any psychotic symptoms or was brief in duration, relative to the duration of the psychotic symptoms in A.

E. Onset of illness before age 45.

F. Not due to any organic mental disorder or mental retardation.

Subtypes Meet Criteria for Schizophrenia Plus

Disorganized Type

A. Schizophrenia.

B. Frequent incoherence.

C. Absence of systematized delusions.
D. Affect blunted, inappropriate or silly (generally, hebephrenic patients classified here).

Catatonic Type

A. Schizophrenia.
B. Throughout the active period of the current episode of illness, the clinical picture is dominated by any of the following:
  (1) Catatonic stupor or mutism (marked decrease in reactivity to environment and/or reduction of spontaneous movements and activity.)
  (2) Catatonic rigidity (maintains a rigid posture against efforts to move him).
  (3) Catatonic excitement (apparently purposeless and stereotyped excited motor activity, not influenced by external stimuli).
  (4) Catatonic posturing (voluntary assumption of inappropriate or bizarre posture).

Paranoid Type

A. Schizophrenia.
B. In active period, clinical picture dominated by one or more of the following:
  (1) Persecutory delusions.
  (2) Grandiose delusions.
  (3) Delusion of jealousy.
  (4) Hallucinations with a persecutory or grandiose content.

Undifferentiated Type

A. Schizophrenia.
B. Psychotic symptoms prominent.
C. Not meet criteria of other subtypes.

Residual Type

A. Once had an episode of schizophrenia.
B. Now no prominent psychotic symptoms.
C. Still shows signs such as blunted or inappropriate affect, eccentric behavior, social withdrawal or communication disorder.

Paranoid Disorders

Diagnostic Criteria

A. Persistent persecutory delusions or delusions of jealousy is the predominant clinical feature.
B. Does not have any of the symptoms of criterion A of Schizophrenia, such as bizarre delusions (content is patently absurd).
C. No evidence of incoherence, marked loosening of associations or prominent hallucinations.
D. Emotion and behavior are appropriate to content of the delusional system.
E. The full depressive or manic syndrome (criteria A and B of Depressive or Manic Episode) is either not present, or if present, developed well after any psychotic symptoms.
F. Duration of illness at least one week from onset of a noticeable change.
G. Not due to organic mental disorder.

Paranoia Type

Diagnostic Criteria
A. Paranoid Disorder.
B. A chronic and simple persecutory delusional system of at least 6 months duration.
C. No evidence of incoherence, marked loosening of associations or prominent hallucinations.
D. Emotion and behavior are appropriate to the delusional system.
E. A Shared Paranoid Disorder.

Shared Type

A. Paranoid disorder.
B. Delusion system shared with a previously paranoid psychotic.

Acute Paranoid Type

Same as Paranoia except duration under 6 months.

Atypical Paranoid Disorder (Residual Category)

Schizoaffective Disorders

A. Has depressive and/or manic symptoms of at least 1-week duration.

B. Has Type A symptoms of schizophrenia in the context of an affective disorder.
C. A syndrome overlapping temporally with B. A must precede or develop at the same time as B.
D. Duration at least one week.
E. Not Organic Mental Disorder.

Schizopheneform

Same criteria as Schizophrenia except duration of illness (prodromal, active residual) more than 1 week, less than 6 months.

Brief Reactive Psychoses

A. Symptoms in B follow stress or
B. At least one of the following:
    (1) Incoherence, derailment, or marked illogical thinking.
    (2) Delusions.
    (3) Hallucinations.
    (4) Grossly disorganized or catatonic behavior.
C. Duration more than a few hours, but less than 1 week.
D. Not preceded by a period of increasing psychopathology.
E. Not organic.

Atypical Psychoses (Residual Category)

Subtypes of Schizophrenia

We will initially focus on the more common subtypes: process, paranoid, and schizoaffective.

Process Schizophrenia

Early childhood onset does not refer to sensitive, neurotic, inhibited or shy children, but to those with obvious psychiatric difficulties. These children are peculiar, asocial, ostracized, cold and deviant. Their school records are poor. When admitted to hospitals, their speech is barely intelligible. They appear evasive, vague, guarded and perplexed. Their behavior may be bizarre for many years, before gradually deteriorating into an overt schizophrenic break. Schizophrenics with childhood asociality (sometimes called process schizophrenics) have a poor prognosis. There are many schemes for the subtyping of schizophrenia (e.g., chronic schizophrenia or schizophrenia of poor prognosis). It can be derived from the fact that chronicity has developed; process or childhood asociality denotes that chronicity is anticipated, while emphasizing the asocial childhood history. A detailed consideration of this scheme is beyond the scope of this book, but we would stress that this dimension is a common feature of most schemes and is backed by research data.

There are several predictors of poor prognosis: an early onset, a gradual onset, and childhood asociality. In addition, the initial response to treatment predicts a long-term prognosis, i.e., a patient who has had several schizophrenic episodes and who may remit slightly, but does not remit fully, has a bad prognosis over the long term. The various diagnostic schemes emphasize one or the other of these prognostic indicators, but they are all interrelated.

The converse has a good prognosis: a normal childhood with a late age of onset, which is acute, and complete recovery from the initial episode. This is classically considered reactive schizophrenia or schizophrenia with a good prognosis.

Paranoid Schizophrenia

The predominant symptoms are persistent persecutory or grandiose delusions or hallucinations. In addition, there may be delusions of jealousy. Typically these patients have angry outbursts, periods of fear, delusions of reference, and are often preoccupied over concerns of autonomy, gender identity and sexual preference.

Before treatment these patients are often guarded, noncommunicative, and agitated. However, the impairment in functioning may be minimal if the symptoms have not been acted upon, and gross disorganization is relatively rare with these patients. Similarly, their affective responsiveness seems preserved and appropriate. Yet, sometimes, when their suspicions are allayed, they speak rapidly and directly, hoping to gain an ally. Often they believe their delusions to be real and may deny that they themselves are ill.

Schizoaffective Schizophrenia

Patients can be be hyperactive and angry, or depressed and retarded upon admission. The onset of illness is often abrupt. Initially, they may appear to be manic depressive. But gross Kraepelinian signs including perceptual and cognitive disorder follow soon after. Bizarre mannerisms and postures, distorted thinking, persecutory delusions and hallucinations, extreme reference ideas and blatant social misinterpretations can be expected to occur.

Patients often have premorbid histories of being outgoing, sociable and capable. If you examine their childhood histories with a critical eye, you can of course find problems. Also, you must realize that it is difficult to imagine any person or family so absolutely normal that close examination could not turn up some difficulties.

This subgroup reacts more favorably to psychotropic drug treatment and exhibits the most successful longterm outcome.

We are enthusiastic about the importance of psychotherapeutic intervention with patients and their families. Since these patients appear to be well-adjusted, capable, and functioning members of society before they became ill, they often recover completely. Many psychiatrists classify these patients as having an affective illness and there is beginning to be a body of knowledge to support this.

► **Schizophrenic patients often have symptoms of** ◄
various subtypes.

No biochemical tests exist for either schizophrenia itself or its subtypes. These patients often show mixed features: in fact, many patients are diagnosed as "undifferentiated." Since subtypes have prognostic implications, the category "undifferentiated schizophrenia" does not convey much information.

We feel that one should avoid making the diagnosis of undifferentiated schizophrenia and try instead to arrive at the closest approximation to some meaningful category. There are six basic dimensions of schizophrenia (i.e., the presence or absence of childhood asociality, rapid or insidious onset, presence of precipitants, paranoid-nonparanoid and schizoaffective-nonschizoaffective dimensions and the initial response to treatment) which should be considered.

In summary, take the natural history of the patient's illness and use this information for diagnosing the current symptoms.

ONCE DIAGNOSED, SHOULD ALL SCHIZOPHRENICS BE MEDICATED?

Psychiatrists Disagree

Essentially, all double-blind drug studies using adequate dosage show that acute schizophrenic decompensation terminates more rapidly and completely with antipsychotic medication. Most psychiatrists agree that antipsychotic drugs should be used to terminate schizophrenic psychosis; however, exceptions exist.

Some authorities, such as R. D. Laing, believe drug treatment to be undesirable because it robs the patient of the psychotic experience. According to Laing, the psychotic patient gains knowledge of himself and others as he reaches out from his autistic world via his acute illness. Yet, regardless of his theoretical opinion, Laing and his coworkers report using antipsychotic medication in treating a great many of their patients (Esterson et al., 1965).

Psychiatrists may seem to disagree in principle, but they may, in fact, agree when discussing individual patients.

It is important that diagnostic arguments not be merely semantic disputes over the definition of terms. For example, a biologically oriented psychiatrist might diagnose patient A as a chronic schizophrenic and prescribe phenothiazines and diagnose patient B as having a hysterical psychosis and prescribe psychotherapy. A psychoanalytic psychiatrist might feel that the same patient A has some sort of organic process and prescribe drugs, and call patient B a schizophrenic and treat him with psychotherapy. Assuming that patients A and B respond to their respective treatments, we would then have two psychiatrists treating patients in the same fashion, but drawing opposite conclusions about the treatment of "schizophrenia." Unfortunately, there is no ultimate diagnostic test and psychiatrists vary greatly in their definition of schizophrenia. The example above is not far-fetched and is demonstrated by Sullivan who describes what we would call early onset chronic schizophrenia as an essentially organic condition, distinct from schizophrenia. It is relevant to paraphrase Sullivan on this point:

Before I present my own views on schizophrenia let me say something about simple dementia praecox which I do not include among the schizophrenic illnesses. There are some people, perhaps at the age of 14, 15, or 16...In general these people simply gradually fall apart in a sort of caricature of a regression. They eventually reach a deteriorated state which is reminiscent of the late condition in hebephrenia. I believe these people suffer from some kind of organic deterioration. I have seen a few of them and wasted some time with some of them...Here we may have a hereditarily determined deterioration...On the basis of this sort of experience simple dementia praecox may be deleted from the schizophrenic illness so far as I am concerned. (Sullivan, 1956).

Parenthetically, it is of interest to add that Sullivan (1931) describes the concept of process and reactive schizophrenia, noting the poor prognosis of patients who had an insidious onset in a review of 100 cases seen at Sheppard and Enoch Pratt Hospital. Sullivan considers what organically oriented psychiatrists diagnose as schizophrenia as dementia praecox, an organic condition which may be hereditary.

Although opinions about therapy tend to polarize (for example, drug psychiatrists against psychoanalytic psychiatrists), we do not think that these polarized positions are useful. We are convinced that appropriate psychological intervention with the patient, his family and their problems is important in helping the patient cope with his present illness, achieve his potential and avoid relapse. Furthermore, it is essential to deal with the patient and his psychological problems in a human manner. Nevertheless, pharmacological treatments in cases where drugs are indicated are helpful and can be handled humanely. The components of a combined psychological and pharmacological approach, rather than interfering, may actually complement each other. In Chapter 2, we review studies comparing and contrasting drug and social treatments, but, for most schizophrenic patients, both should be used.

There is no doubt that drug treatment has made an important difference in the fate of schizophrenics. Prior to 1955 when drugs were introduced in the United States, the population of patients in state mental hospitals had been rising substantially over the years. Following the use of these drugs, the number of patients hospitalized has dropped dramatically (Fig. 1.2).

Schizotypical Personality Disorders: To Medicate or Not to Medicate?

There is considerable evidence that antipsychotic drugs are effective in treating overt schizophrenics with blatant psychotic symptoms, and that manifest hallucinations, delusions, extreme

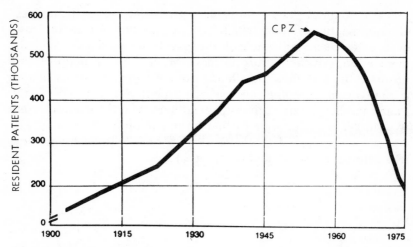

Figure 1.2. Inpatient population of state and county mental hospitals.

withdrawal and bizarre mannerisms sharply diminish with medication. The improvement can be easily monitored even by a layman who lacks special knowledge. In contrast, schizotypical personality disorders (latent schizophrenics) simple schizophrenics, borderline personalities, and other such diagnoses create problems for psychopharmacologists. As far as we know, there exist no controlled double-blind studies or extensive clinical experience which has evaluated the use of antipsychotic drugs in these diagnostic categories. Since psychopharmacology is based upon great changes in overtly manifested symptoms, the technology for measuring change is based on easily observable behaviors. Newer methods must be developed for dealing with more subtle alterations. Many clinicians regard the diagnosis of the borderline state as useful. Research in this area of psychopharmacology has lagged behind, and because of the inherent difficulty in measuring the borderline state, no information is available about using medication with such patients. Clinical experience indicates that antipsychotic medication is helpful for some borderline patients, but firm data is lacking.

Our Conclusion

We favor vigorous psychological and pharmacological treatment for most schizophrenic patients. Treating an overtly psychotic patient often involves dealing with colorful and florid primary process material. The results are interesting, affect-laden psychotherapeutic sessions, which may or may not be fruitful. However, after resolving much of the psychosis with antipsychotic medication, psychotherapy is more orderly and probably more useful to the patient, although less dramatic to an observer behind a one-way mirror. The purpose of psychotherapy is the former. Pharmacotherapy potentiates psychotherapy; it does not interfere with it. We will elaborate further on this point later on.

(For references, see end of Chapter 2.)

chapter TWO

Choosing an Antipsychotic

CONSIDER THESE FACTORS BEFORE DRUG TREATMENT BEGINS

History, Physical and Laboratory Examinations

A Drug-Free Interval

Observations and diagnoses of patients should be made during a drug-free period so that if medication is warranted the most beneficial drug with the fewest side effects can be selected. These observations also aid in distinguishing false from true side effects after chemotherapy has begun. Some institutions have made at least a 48-hour, drug-free interval a standard procedure for most patients who begin drug treatment. There are, of course, patients who are so severely ill that immediate emergency treatment is indicated.

The Patient's History

The psychiatrist must note any medical condition that may be aggravated by drug intake. An important part of the patient's history includes the somatic therapies the patient and his close relatives have received.

Previous adverse reactions to psychoactive drugs, as well as any other medicines being taken that might cause harmful interaction, should be specifically noted.

The history must include a careful attempt to elicit symptoms that later could be falsely attributed to a psychoactive agent and to administer a side effects checklist before drug therapy. Symptoms such as dizziness, headaches, motor disturbances, dry mouth, gastrointestinal discomfort, constipation, tremor, restlessness, der-

19

matitis and visual disturbances are often erroneously attributed to psychoactive agents. Such symptoms may, in fact, be manifestations of a psychiatric illness.

The Physical and Laboratory Examinations

Record blood pressure in hospitalized patients, not only during admission excitement, but also later when the patient is calm. A drop in blood pressure might otherwise be erroneously attributed to drug intake. One double-blind study found a 25% incidence of postural hypotension in a placebo group.

When possible, record both recumbent and standing blood pressures before starting medication.

The patient's gait must be carefully observed to distinguish the patient's predrug walk, often peculiar, from a drug-induced parkinsonism. This precaution extends to other abnormal movements as well.

Just as a patient who sees a new doctor for the first time has a screening physical and a laboratory examination, a patient who starts on antipsychotic medication often undergoes the same screening procedure for the same reason, namely, to discover any other undiagnosed disease. On rare occasions, an organic etiology underlies an apparent schizophrenic reaction, so that a physical examination will prove useful in this regard. It also provides a baseline against which to evaluate side effects. It is important to note that most of the same rationale for a screening physical and laboratory examination also applies to schizophrenics who are treated *without* drugs.

Cooperation

In pharmacotherapy, as in psychotherapy, a therapeutic alliance between the patient and the physician must be established whenever possible. An agreement must be made between you and your patient to overcome whatever is "sick." The precise reasons for antipsychotic medication must be explained to the patient and his agreement and cooperation won whenever possible.

A clinical example: A 23-year-old unmarried attractive nurse complaining of weight loss, depression, excessive crying and social withdrawal was offered amitriptyline (Elavil) after three hour-long psychiatric interviews. She refused because she did not want to be dependent upon medication for her happiness. A half tablet of dextraoamphetamine (Dexedrine) in the recent past had made her feel too well, and she feared this easy solution. It was then explained to her that she had already been depressed for five months and that amitriptyline would help her more rapidly than psychotherapy. Whether she chose to take the drug or not, she had psychosocial problems that she would have to overcome with a therapist, and it was up to her how long she wished to suffer. The patient was then instructed to go home and think it over. On her next visit, she agreed to try amitriptyline.

By explaining that a drug can offer symptomatic relief, but not solve all her problems, and that she will be helped with these difficulties whether she takes the drug or not, the doctor allows the patient some control. In the above case, the decision of whether or not to take the drug was the patient's. Allow the patient to make some decisions concerning medication. This approach is respectful and can often win the patient's cooperation and confidence. Furthermore, it becomes a vital part of the psychotherapeutic interaction.

Regular intake of medication is not always maintained by many outpatients. Often this is not deliberate, but due to forgetfulness or lack of conscientiousness on their part. Relapse often occurs coincidentally with a patient's stopping his drug intake. In some instances, forgetfulness leads to a low enough dose ingestion, even though the regular dosage schedule is adhered to, so that a certain critical limit is passed and relapse results. In other cases, the patient relapses and then, as part of his psychosis, he does not take his medication. In the former instance, a good doctor-patient relationship may lead to a more conscientious attitude toward taking the medication regularly. In the latter instance, if a good relationship exists with the family, they may recognize the failure to take the medication as a sign of an impending difficulty and bring the patient to the psychiatrist quickly to avoid a relapse.

On psychiatric wards, patients will occasionally "cheek" their medication and not actually ingest it, or give their pills to other patients. If the medication is a subject for discussion between the doctor and the patient, it becomes an open issue and can be handled on a psychotherapeutic level, rather than becoming a target for passive resistance or acting out.

Even in the case of an assaultive, uncontrollable schizophrenic, explain that you are requesting the attendants to hold him down and are injecting him with chlorpromazine (Thorazine) because he is out of control, and the drug will help him regain self-mastery. Although the patient may have the delusion that you are trying to kill him, a possibility exists that the rational part of his mind will consider your words. Questioning patients after recovery from such episodes verifies this assumption. In most mental hospitals, it is possible to win patient cooperation in drug taking at least 99% of the time.

The violent patient needing emergency medication intramuscularly (IM) deserves special comment. Most mental patients take their medication voluntarily. Although they may passively resist or complain to their doctor, few actively refuse. In psychiatric wards containing disturbed and acute patients, only rarely does someone who is extremely agitated and violent require emergency intramuscular medication. Do not assume that these patients will not take oral medication; once the necessity is explained, they usually agree to take their medications, especially after further cajoling. Not uncommonly, patients are paranoid about a drug, feeling that it may be lethal, that they are being executed for their sins, or that the hospital attendants are Russian spies.

In the days before tranquilizers, extremely excited patients could exhaust themselves and die. This was sometimes prevented with cold packs, seclusion rooms, or baths, but the patient would nevertheless remain severely psychotic for a long time. Now, after high-dose IM medication, the patient often becomes cooperative by the next morning, although usually with residual schizophrenic symptoms. In extreme excitement, medication can be lifesaving. During violent paranoid delusion, the patient may direct his aggression against persons or property. This can cause serious injury or death to other patients or toward personnel. IM medication can dramatically relieve such violent behavior. Acute episodes usually have a good prognosis, so it is not uncommon to have a patient remit from his schizophrenic episode and leave the hospital in several weeks—as an essentially normal person. When extreme excitement and violence occur, they often do not erupt instantly. Rather, the patient becomes progressively more excited, sometimes over several minutes or hours. Thus, you should intervene earlier rather than later.

A vicious circle ensues when a patient becomes violent and excitable. He suffers extremes of arousability and violence, while perceiving himself as losing control of his own impulses and aggressions. This loss of control is extremely frightening and anxiety-provoking; the patient sees himself changing into a raving maniac. This high-level anxiety completes the circle, which in turn increases the hostility and violence. The fear of becoming violent is so frightening that it tends to push the patient further into psychosis. Once patients get into this vicious circle, they commonly escalate the violence, often within hours. Intervene early, in spite of any reluctance to give disagreeable intramuscular medication or to place the patient in seclusion. If medication is delayed the patient becomes even more frightened and, therefore, harder to control. If you procrastinate and the patient becomes violent, when he recovers (and these individuals often make complete recoveries), he will have disturbing memories of his destructive acts. For example, if a patient in such a violent episode blinds a nursing assistant and then recovers several weeks later, he has to live with the knowledge that he caused harm to another human being.

If you later talk to patients about such episodes, they report feeling themselves losing control and welcome the physician who takes a firm hand. They are grateful for your preventing them from doing something that they would later regret. It is like caring for a patient who has passed out. Almost every normal person would wish, if he were found unconscious, that a physician would take the necessary measures to diagnose and treat his illness. The physician, in taking care of the unconscious patient, should make this same assumption. Similarly, the physician can act as an agent with the violent patient who, in his normal state, would want his extreme aggression controlled.

Listening to patients' ideas, attitudes and theories about the intended medication helps you win their cooperation. One patient on the ward protested that a drug offered to him was ineffective for one of his friends and produced a bad side effect in a second. His unwillingness to take the medication can only be understood in this context.

The psychiatrist must understand his own unconscious psychological reaction to the way a patient asks for a drug. The patient who too eagerly wants medication and expects magic relief can make the physician question whether to dispense it. For example, a depressed elderly woman *should* be given the medication she wants for her headaches and upset stomach, despite her constant begging and her magical beliefs that this will cure her symptoms. You must recognize when a patient's repeated demanding makes you angry and desirous of withholding the magic pill.

We have chosen an example in which the physician might gratify a reasonable request from the patient. You could easily choose examples when he should withhold unnecessary medication. The point is that you must be aware of your own feelings toward the request and deal with them appropriately. The patient's feelings about medication and the feelings induced in the doctor can furnish valuable material for discussion in psychotherapy.

A medication-therapeutic alliance is important. It assures that the patient will continue to take the drug after discharge. Even during hospitalization, but particularly as outpatients, one-third to one-half of psychiatric patients do not take their prescribed medication. Many patients, once discharged, require maintenance therapy. Only if you win their cooperation will they continue to take these expensive medications.

The cooperation of others besides the doctor and patient must be considered. The family must be convinced that drug therapy is worth the expense; they may have to be involved in making certain that the patient takes the drug, especially during relapse when he wishes to take less or none at all, but in fact requires more.

In the hospital, various staff members are often at odds over medication. Generally, social workers and psychologists are negative toward drugs, while doctors, nurses and attendants are strongly in favor of medication. Nurses and attendants spend the most time with the patients and, thus, have the greatest need for them to be nonpsychotic. Social workers and psychologists are not involved in drug administration and spend less time with patients.

The nurse who actually administers the drug may not be in total agreement with a doctor's orders; she may, in fact, give too little or too much since she is the sole interpreter of the doctor's drug orders. Clinical examples show an occasional discrepancy between the psychiatrist's orders and what the nurse actually dispenses to the patient.

Finally, the doctor himself must undergo an analysis of his own drug attitudes. Many physicians who value self-reliance and independence view drugs negatively as a crutch and unreasonably withhold them from patients. An example of this phenomenon has been recently shown in a fine teaching medical hospital: narcotics were withheld from patients in extreme pain. You must always maintain a clear perspective—drugs are *not* the entire answer, but a useful tool in a total therapy.

Administering a Drug in the Private Psychiatric Office

Strictly analytic psychiatrists who do not touch or examine their patients probably should not prescribe drugs, since they are unable to adequately monitor pulse, blood pressure and neurological, dermatological, ocular, oral or other side effects, and, thus, are reluctant to use sufficiently large and effective dosage. Such physicians should send their patients to a drug-oriented psychiatrist who should see the patient on a regular basis for regulation of dosage and monitoring of side effects. Repeated use of the same consultant enables the two physicians to work constructively together for the benefit of the patient and to minimize problems of physician competition, communication, splitting of the transference, and dosage adjustment designed to maximize pharmacological effect and avoid side effects

References

Appleton, W. S.: Third psychoactive drug usage guide. Dis. Nerv. Syst. 37(1): 39–51, January 1976.
A short outline of the whole field.

Appleton, W. S.: Legal problems in psychiatric drug prescription. Am. J. Psychiatry 124: 877–882, 1968.
Covers the package insert, informed consent, physical examination, suicidal patients and drug experiment.

Axelrod, J.: Neurotransmitters. Scient. Am. 230 (6): 58–71, 1974.
Very clear, helpful, illustrated, brief and accurate.

Ayd, F. J.: International Drug Therapy Newsletter. [Published monthly (now bimonthly) since January 1966.]
A thorough and excellent review of what is new and also of old issues. An excellent aid in keeping up.

Baldessarini, R. J.: Chemotherapy in Psychiatry. Cambridge, Mass., Harvard University Press, 1977.
A brief and excellent overview.
Biological Therapies in Psychiatry.
From the Massachusetts General Hospital. (Similar to the Ayd newsletter; also excellent).

Central NP Research Laboratory, Veterans Administration Hospital, Perry Point, Maryland, Staff: Drug Treatment in Psychiatry. Washington, U. S. Government Printing Office, 1970.
An excellent review, brief and helpful.

Cooper, J. R., Bloom, F. E., and Roth, R. H.: The Biochemical Basis of Neuropharmacology, 3rd ed. New York, Oxford University Press, 1977.
A brief, scholarly, magnificent introduction and guide to this complex area.

Corbett, L.: Clinical differentiation of

the schizophrenic and affective disorders: A comparison of the bleulerian and phenomenologic approaches to diagnosis. In *Psychiatric Diagnosis: Explanation of Biological Predictions*, edited by H. Akiskal and W. Webb. New York, Medical & Scientific Books, 1978.

DiMascio, A., and Shader, R. I., eds.: *Butyrophenones in Psychiatry*. New York, Raven Press, 1972.
Thorough, excellent, brief monograph.

Esterson, A., Cooper, D., and Laing, R.: Results of family-oriented therapy with hospitalized schizophrenia. Br. Med. J. 11: 1462–1465, 1965.

Freedman, A., Kaplan, H., and Sadock, B.: *Modern Synopsis of Comprehensive Textbook of Psychiatry II*. Williams & Wilkins, Baltimore, 1977.

Hollister, L. E.: *Clinical Use of Psychotherapeutic Drugs*. Springfield Ill., Charles C Thomas, 1973.
An excellent book.

Honigfeld, G.: Non-specific factors in treatment. 1. Review of placebo reactions and placebo reactors. Dis. Nerv. Syst. 25: 145–156, March 1964.

Honigfeld, G.: Non-specific factors in treatment. 2. Review of social psychological factors, Dis. Nerv. Syst. 25: 225–239, April 1964.
These two articles are still the best on the subject.

Johnston, H., and Holzman, P.: *Assessing Schizophrenic Thinking*. Jossey-Bass, San Francisco, 1979.

Klein, D. F. and Davis, J.: *Diagnosis and Drug Treatment of Psychiatric Disorders*. Baltimore, Williams and Wilkins, 1969.

A 480-page aging giant, still indispensable. High quality in-depth coverage with excellent bibliography.

Klein, D. F., and Gittleman-Klein, R.: *Progress in Psychiatric Drug Treatment*. New York, Brunner/Mazel, Vol. 1, 1975, Vol. 2, 1976.
Reprints of the major papers of the year.

Lipton, M. A., DiMascio, A., and Killam, K. F., eds.: *Psychopharmacology: A Generation of Progress*. New York, Raven Press, 1978.
A 1731-page magnificent, in-depth review of the field.

May, P. R. A.: *Treatment of Schizophrenia: A Comparative Study of Five Treatment Methods*. New York, Science House, 1968.
A classic study supporting the use of drugs in schizophrenia.

Mayer-Gross, W., Slater, E., and Roth, M.: *Clinical Psychiatry*, Baltimore, Williams & Wilkins, 1969.

Shader, R. I., ed.: *Manual of Psychiatric Therapeutics: Pratical Psychopharmacology and Psychiatry*. Boston, Little, Brown and Co., 1975.
Although there are many contributors the quality is uniformly high. Theory and practice are covered.

Shader, R. I.: *Psychiatric Complications of Medical Drugs*. New York, Raven Press, 1972.
Still the best review book on this subject.

Sullivan, H. S.: *Clinical Studies in Psychiatry*. W. W. Norton, New York, 1956.

Wing, J.: *Present State Examination*, 9th ed. Institute of Psychiatry, 1971.

chapter THREE

Principles of Prescribing Antipsychotics

The major goal in prescribing an antipsychotic drug is reducing the psychosis. This reduction is monitored by symptomatic changes. Specify your therapeutic goal, such as:
- Eliminating hallucinations.
- Improving socialization.
- Decreasing hyperactivity.
- Improving self-care.
- Eliminating assaultiveness.

Since all the antipsychotics are similar in therapeutic efficacy, and have the same range and side effects, we will first discuss the therapeutic use of the antipsychotics as a class, then comment on the differences in side effects among members of this class and then go on to discuss side effects in detail.

Dosage must be increased gradually until a therapeutic dose is achieved, or until a rare and serious side effect occurs. No standard dose exists. Different patients require different doses for optimal therapeutic effect. The correct dose must be determined empirically (Table 3.1).

Increase the dose gradually, because patients differ substantially in how well they tolerate antipsychotic drugs. Acute schizophrenics can ingest large quantities. Elderly patients with organic brain damage do well on much smaller amounts.

In treating schizophrenic patients, you can safely use higher than necessary doses, since only rarely do serious side effects actually occur. The majority of those that do are not dose-related. Furthermore, the patient may not be helped when treated with lower doses. For this reason, overshooting the optimal dose and then reducing it is a better policy than never achieving the optimal

Table 3.1
Dosage Equivalency (Approximate)

Ratio (to Thorazine)	Drug	Dose in mg (equalling 100 mg Thorazine)
1:1	Thorazine	100
2:1	Sparine	200
1:3	Vesprin	30
1:5	Tindal	20
1:50	Prolixin	2
1:10	Trilafon	10
1:6	Compazine	16
1:3	Proketazine	30
1:20	Stelazine	5
1:8	Dartal	12
1:10	Repoise	10
1:1	Mellaril	100
1:6	Quide	10
1:2	Serentil	50
1:2	Taractan	50
1:30	Navane	3
1:10	Moban	10
1:50	Haldol	2
1:10	Loxitane	10
1:200	Prolixin decanoate or enanthate	0.5–0.7

level. We will comment first on dosage for the average schizophrenic patient.

THE AVERAGE DAILY DOSE

For acute schizophrenics this amount is usually between 400
and 900 phenothiazine units (i.e., Thorazine, between 400 and 900
mg; Stelazine, between 10 and 40 mg; Prolixin, between 6 and 18
mg; Haldol, between 8 and 40 mg; Loxapine, between 60 and 100
mg [see Table 3.5].

How rapidly this 400- to 900-unit level is reached depends upon
the patient's age, size, weight, previous drug history and behavior.
The average acute antipsychotic dose is about 600 units (chlorpromazine equivalent) for a healthy patient.

Age. The older the patient, the less phenothiazine is required to
achieve a therapeutic goal.

Size and Weight. Obviously, small, frail patients are able to
tolerate less.

Previous Drug History. The capacity to have both required and tolerated large drug doses in the past greatly influences current drug treatment. Heavy smokers also require larger doses.

Behavior. Some behaviors require much more urgent medication than others, especially assaultive behaviors in open-door hospitals.

RAPID NEUROLEPTIZATION—INTRAMUSCULAR

Intramuscular neuroleptics are being used more and more for aggressive, combative, destructive and excited psychotic patients to protect them and others from the dangers of their unrestrained behavior and to avoid or minimize hospitalization. A small IM test dose can be given if the situation is not critical. The following possible causes should first be ruled out: head injuries, space-occupying lesions, epilepsy, severe hyper- and hypotension, anticholinergic intoxication and electrolyte imbalance.

A piperazine phenothiazine, thiothixene, haloperidol or Loxapine is most often used parenterally in the psychiatric emergency because little or no injection site pain, excessive sedation, or cardiovascular side effects occur. Neuroleptics are best injected into the deltoid in the following initial IM doses:

Perphenazine, 10 mg—range 4-30 mg
Trifluoroperazine, 3 mg—range 1-10 mg
Fluphenazine, 2.5 mg—range 1-25 mg
Haloperidol, 2 mg—range 1-10 mg
Thiothixene, 5 mg—range 4-30 mg

We suggest that a PRN (i.e., as needed) order for an IM parkinsonian agent be written for the patient in the event of an extrapyramidal reaction.

Subsequent IM or PO dose, if required, should be given hourly (in occasional cases after 30 minutes) while the blood pressure is monitored. Most patients are asleep or adequately medicated within six hours and require about 20-60 mg of fluphenazine during the first 24 hours. The oral dose prescribed for the second 24 hours should be one to one and one half times that required IM in the first 24. It is administered in liquid form for several days before being switched to tablet. Night time sleep (6 to 7 hours) is used as a monitor of improvement and the dosage is gradually reduced to that which can be lowest while still being effective.

Interpersonal factors often play a prominent role in violent episodes or cases of extreme excitement. You must work them out after the patient is under control. Indeed, once the situation is controlled by pharmacotherapy, the tension level on the ward often goes down markedly. Fruitful discussion of the interpersonal relationships that may have stirred up the patient can now take place: "Put out the fire and then worry about fire prevention."

STAGES IN PHENOTHIAZINE TREATMENT OF ACUTE SCHIZOPHRENIA

Heinz Lehmann differentiated four treatment stages, each to be achieved within a definite time span. Failure to do so indicates inadequate dosage or the use of the wrong drug. The four stages are:

1. Medicated cooperation—Within 1 to 5 days, the patient should no longer be in a stage of motor excitement and hyperactivity should cease.

2. Socialization—Within 2 days to two months, the patient should participate in ward activities, even though his thought disorder continues.

3. Elimination of thought disorder—This occurs last, often not before 1 to 6 weeks.

4. Maintenance therapy.

Figures 3.1 and 3.2 show the average improvement rates of acute schizophrenic patients from several studies. Some patients improve dramatically over a few days. Others improve gradually over a few months. The stages through which improvement occurs—cooperation, socialization, elimination of thought disorder—are somewhat variable. Stages are not always clearly defined.

The stages described by Lehmann have not yet been verified by controlled research. We feel that "stages" is an improper conceptualization of this phenomena. In our opinion, the drugs effect cooperation, socialization and thought disorder from the outset, so that all of the phases, in essence, start in the beginning. What differs is when they end. If a patient is in an acute psychotic decompensation, the first problem in his management is the restoration of some degree of self-control so that he can minimally cooperate, take care of his own body functions, not exhaust himself with hyperactivity, and not be violent against himself or others. Whether or not the patient has thought disorder is really not a critical problem at this time. Extremely disturbed patients

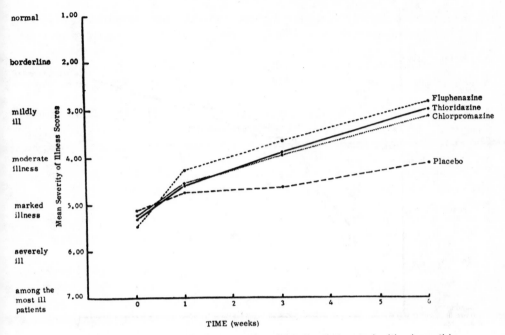

Figure 3.1. Severity of illness over time in patients treated with phenothiazines. (Data from NIMH-PSC Collaborative Study I)

cannot socialize, so this poses no difficulty. After the initial emergency has passed, the therapeutic task turns to the resocialization of the patient. Empirically, the thought disorder seems to persist for a prolonged period of time, so that a patient can be socializing on the ward reasonably well, but still have some residual thought disorder. Whether subsequent research will verify the exact phases as Lehmann describes them remains to be seen. If his ideas are not taken too literally, we do feel in some sense that some patients do progress through these problem areas, and that it may be a useful way to think about the process of reintegration of the psychotic patient.

THE PHENOTHIAZINE LAG PERIOD

Oddly enough, scientific articles and package inserts describing antidepressant drugs and lithium refer to a lag period of between five days and three weeks. However, a phenothiazine lag period is

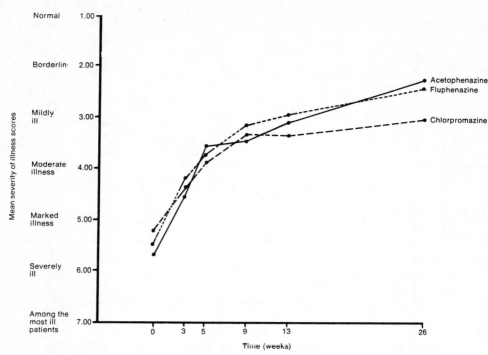

Figure 3.2. Severity of illness over time in patients treated with phenothiazines. (Data from NIMH-PSC Collaborative Study II)

never mentioned. Certainly one exists. Anyone who has used these drugs knows that instantaneous results simply do not occur.

We wish to propose a formal heading "antipsychotic lag period," in order to encourage psychiatrists to wait more patiently for the therapeutic effect, and to discourage raising the dose too rapidly to achieve a desired result. The time course of the antipsychotic drugs is given in Figure 3.1.

Refrain from elevating the dose too rapidly, even with disturbed patients. Six hundred units of chlorpromazine equivalents should be adequate for many patients during the initial 24-hour period. An occasional elevation to 1000 mg may be made. Once 1500 mg daily is reached, only rarely does additional improvement occur from further dosage elevation. Because a rare patient benefits from up to 4000 mg, the 1500 mg ceiling is not absolute, but should be exceeded only in unusual circumstances.

With the exception of thioridazine, there is no upper limit to any antipsychotic in absolute terms. Chlorpromazine, because of its high sedating properties, has its upper limit determined to some degree by the behavioral end point of excessive sedation. If one pools information from double-blind studies, the mean dose of chlorpromazine in the acute treatment phase is about 750 mg. With chlorpromazine, it is not infrequently necessary to treat some patients with twice the usual dose, or up to 1500 mg, to deal with a particularly difficult psychotic problem. On the other hand, with fluphenazine, 10 mg is roughly the equivalent of 800 mg of chlorpromazine, and it is no problem at all to go to 20 mg because the upper antipsychotic dose is not limited by excessive sedation. Indeed, some investigators have gone to 10 times, or even 100 times this figure (1000 mg of fluphenazine) without interference from alarming side effects. Certainly the incidence of side effects is only slightly higher in patients on 1200 mg of fluphenazine vs. 30 mg. We would emphasize the importance of adjusting the dose in accordance with its effects on the individual patient, and definitely would not encourage these high dose levels in any but exceptional patients. We recognize that high doses are needed in treating the resistant patient, and further discussion concerning high dose treatment will follow later.

CAN THE ANTIPSYCHOTIC LAG PERIOD BE SHORTENED BY A DIGITALIZING DOSE?

As can be seen from Figures 3.1 and 3.2, patients improve gradually with antipsychotic drugs over a period of several weeks and begin to reach optimal improvement by around 6 weeks. One possible reason for this relatively slow rate of improvement may be that insufficient quantities of the drug reach the receptor to produce the therapeutic effect. If this is the case, the use of a high dose, a so-called digitalizing or loading dose, in the first few days, may allow certain critical drug levels to be reached in the brain and, hence, effect improvement at a much faster rate. Consequently, a high dose administration in the first few days should show a more rapid improvement and possibly lead to better results after three weeks. In our group, we tested this hypothesis by randomly assigning acute decompensated schizophrenics to two groups: Our group received a standard (high normal) dose of haloperidol (15 mg/day p.o.) for 21 days, and the other group received a double-blind digitalizing dose (60 mg/day for 5 days intramuscularly). This was slowly tapered and ended at a 15 mg oral dose on day 21. The results are shown in Figure 3.3. It can be seen that patients on the digitalizing dose did not do better than patients on the standard dose. It would seem that, on the average, digitalizing the patient with an initial high dose does not produce any better results than the standard treatment, when an adequate dose is given. Some studies have compared a large initial dose against a very small initial dose and found that the very small initial dose produced less favorable results. We feel it is important that the dosage in the initial period be adequate.

Given that patients metabolize these drugs at different rates, and have different plasma levels, one must adjust the dose to a patient's clinical response. Some patients clinically do require high doses during the initial phase. What this study indicates is that all patients do not show improvement with a digitalizing dose. The digitalizing dose produced a higher prevalence of side effects, such as dystonias, so that it is not a completely innocuous procedure. However, it did not produce dangerous side effects, such as severe postural hypotension.

IF THE PHENOTHIAZINE IS INEFFECTIVE

Is the patient actually taking the drug? So many hospitalized patients do not take their medication that this may always remain

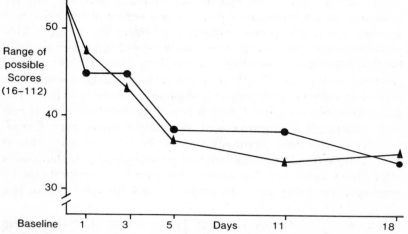

Figure 3.3. Brief psychiatric rating scale—total. ●, Standard dose; ▲, loading dose.

a suspicion. You may have to examine the mouth for a cheeked tablet or administer the drug in liquid form. After 15 days at adequate dosage, if no effect is observed in an acute schizophrenic, change to another antipsychotic drug.

Of course such a suggestion is arbitrary, and in a patient who is doing poorly, one should switch earlier. If a patient is doing moderately well, you may not necessarily decide at 15 days that switching is in order, but may do so at a later time. Experienced clinicians do note that, occasionally, a patient will respond to one antipsychotic but not to another. The mechanism for this has not been worked out, but it is important to vary both dose and type of medication to achieve an optimal response with minimal side effects.

MAINTENANCE THERAPY

After inpatients have remitted from the acute psychotic phase and have substantially improved, the question arises as to the duration of the drug treatment on a maintenance basis. A review of the literature shows that there have been 29 properly controlled, double-blind studies in both Europe and the United States; every one has shown an important difference in terms of the rate of relapses between those patients who have been given antipsychotic medication and those who were placed on placebo (Table 3.2).

Hogarty, Goldberg and their collaborators have performed a particularly important evaluation of maintenance phenothiazine treatment on 374 chronic schizophrenics who were discharged after recovery from their illness. After a stabilization period on maintenance phenothiazine, half these patients were assigned to maintenance chlorpromazine and half to placebo. Half of each group attended psychotherapeutic sessions consisting of individual case work and vocational rehabilitation counseling. Thus, we are able to compare maintenance phenothiazines and psychological intervention in the four possible combinations. The results were as follows: after one year, 73% of the placebo patients without psychotherapy had relapsed; 63% of the placebo plus psychotherapy patients had relapsed; 33% of the drug maintenance group relapsed; 26% of the drug maintenance plus psychotherapy group relapsed. The data support a substantial drug-placebo difference. Overall, 31% of the drug-treated group relapsed as compared to

Table 3.2
Antipsychotic Prevention of Relapse*

Study	No. of patients	Relapse on placebo	Relapse on drug	Difference in relapse rate (placebo-drug)
Caffey	259	45%	5%	40%
Prien	762	42%	16%	26%
Prien	325	56%	20%	36%
Schiele	80	60%	3%	57%
Adelson	281	90%	49%	41%
Morton	40	70%	25%	45%
Baro	26	100%	0%	100%
Hershon	62	28%	7%	21%
Rassidakis	84	58%	34%	24%
Melynk	40	50%	0%	50%
Schauver	80	18%	5%	13%
Freeman	86	31%	14%	17%
Whitaker	39	65%	8%	57%
Garfield	27	31%	11%	20%
Diamond	40	70%	25%	45%
Blackburn	53	54%	24%	30%
Gross	109	58%	14%	44%
Englehardt	294	30%	15%	15%
Leff	30	83%	33%	50%
Hogarty	361	67%	31%	36%
Troshinsky	43	63%	4%	59%
Hirsch	74	66%	8%	58%
Chien	31	87%	12%	74%
Gross	61	65%	34%	31%
Rifkin	62	68%	7%	61%
Clark	35	78%	27%	51%
Clark	19	70%	44%	26%
Kinross-Wright	40	70%	5%	65%
Andrews	31	35%	79%	28%
Summary	3519	55%	19%	36%

Summary statistics, $p < 10^{-100}$.

* See J. M. Davis: Overview: Maintenance therapy in psychiatry; I. Schizophrenia. Am J. Psychiatry 132:1237–1245, 1975

68% of the placebo group. Of the patients maintained on active medication, some spontaneously stopped taking their drug. If you do not consider those patients in the drug maintenance group who spontaneously stopped taking their drugs, the relapse rate for these patients, for 12 months, drops to approximately 16%. This, of course, is a marked contrast to a relapse rate of 68% in the placebo group (16% vs. 68%).

Patients on placebo generally relapse at an approximately linear rate, at which time their functioning disintegrates rapidly. They show few schizophrenic symptoms at periodic evaluations until they suddenly become markedly psychotic.

In Figure 3.4, the number of patients not relapsed is plotted vs. time ("semi-log" plot) from two double-blind controlled studies (Caffey et al., 1964; Hogarty and Goldberg, 1974). If a fixed percentage of patients relapse each month, the exponential plot used here corrects for the fact that each month a smaller absolute number of patients have not relapsed and are still in the study.

The data produce an excellent fit to an exponential function, and suggest that *a constant percentage of patients relapse each month*. We were the first to suggest that an exponential function was a good way to think of prophylactic drugs in preventing relapse (Davis, 1976). Expressed this way, the data of Hogarty and Goldberg (1974) indicate that antipsychotic drugs reduced relapses by a factor of 2.5. This is a substantial degree of prophylaxis. These results apply to patients who have a history of chronic relapsing schizophrenia.

Termination of Maintenance. Because of the above disadvantages, you should discontinue maintenance drug therapy whenever possible. Relapse may not become evident for as long as 2 to 3 years. Actually, reports that 50% of the patients relapse are misleading, in the sense that the longer the patient remains off drugs, the greater the percentages of relapse. A more precise way of expressing this point would be to say that the relapse rate for patients with maintenance medication is 2½ times less than that of patients off maintenance medication. Given that about 50% of these patients relapse because they have stopped taking their medication, it may be that the relapse rate would be reduced by 5 times. Thus, the order of magnitude of reduction in relapse is 2½ and, perhaps, even as high as 5. Unfortunately, no way exists to predict which patients will become worse with reduced medication.

The need for continuous therapy should be reviewed periodically. At regular intervals, chronically hospitalized patients should have their medication stopped or their dosage lowered to see if they still need it. This will reduce the incidence of tardive dyskinesia, and an occasional patient will improve once off medication. Stopping long-term maintenance in outpatients is riskier than in those who are institutionalized. One fact emerges from clinical

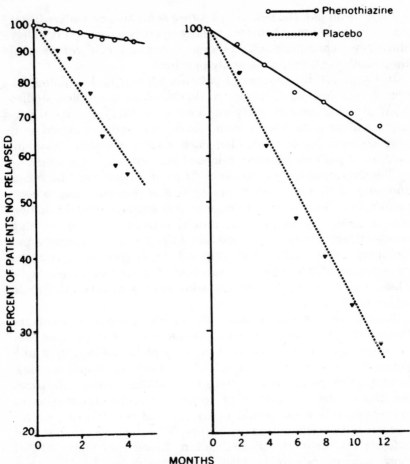

Figure 3.4. Percentage of patients not relapsed on maintenance medication or placebo in two studies. The left-hand portion of the graph shows the percentage of 259 patients who did not relapse on maintenance medication or placebo in a 4-month double-blind controlled study by Caffey and associates (1964). The right-hand portion shows the percentage of 43 patients who did not relapse on maintenance medication or placebo in a 12-month double-blind controlled study by Hogarty and Goldberg (1973). In each case the data were fitted by the method of least squares to an exponential curve.

studies: the greater the dosage required for maintenance, the greater the probability of relapse once the drug is discontinued.

It is of interest that Hogarty (1976) wondered if the rate of relapse, that is the percentage of patients relapsing each month, would be approximately the same several years after the start of the study. When he began to investigate this question, he discovered that only six patients were available for research in the group that initially had received placebo. This is because the relapse rate was so high. There were few unrelapsed patients left after two years. In addition, as with any follow-up study, patients had moved away, which further depleted the sample size. Since drugs decrease the relapse rate substantially, there were a reasonable number of patients in the group that had received maintenance phenothiazine medication. He then discontinued phenothiazines for these patients and observed that the relapse rate, two years after the start of the study, was approximately the same in these patients as it had been for those who had had their drugs discontinued at the start of the study.

The Hogarty and Goldberg group also investigated the social functions of the patients. Patients treated with drugs and psychotherapy did much better in terms of their actual functioning in the community than patients treated with drugs alone. It would appear that "psychotherapy" improves social functions and that the drugs primary effect is to prevent relapses leading to hospitalization. We feel that it is a mistake to think of psychotherapy vs. drugs, and prefer the notion that psychotherapy acts in a manner independent of drugs: drugs act to prevent relapses of schizophrenic illness, whereas psychotherapy acts on psychological social dimensions. Hence, their use is not antagonistic, but rather complementary. Psychotherapy without drugs is ineffective.

Dose

One-half to one-fifth of peak dosage is often used for maintenance. However, there is no standard dose; you must instead arrive at the proper amount empirically for each patient. Minimum drugs for optimal functioning is preferred over an arbitrary maintenance level. Since dosage is often established during hospitalization for acute illness, it tends to remain high. Wary of exacerbation, psychiatrists often fear that if the medication is lowered the patient will not be able to be discharged. You do not have to adminster a maintenance drug more than once a day—just before bedtime seems best. Be sure to adjust the dose downward as the patient improves and eventually to a maintenance dose.

Patient Selection

Patient selection criteria are uncertain. Unfortunately, extended periods (i.e., years) of antipsychotic treatment carry serious risks of tardive dyskinesia. Therefore, reactive psychotics, i.e., those who may have experienced one acute episode with a quick remission in adolescence, may never be ill again, and often do not relapse without medication. Clearly, these patients should *not* be placed on long-term maintenance. Such patients need *not* be treated by long-term chemotherapy, even after a second attack, provided it does not occur too soon after the first. If the acute phase is prolonged, or if the remission is faulty, maintenance medication is indicated. A primary indication for long-term maintenance is the high probability of future relapse. Maintenance therapy in properly selected patients decreases recurrence by at least 250% what would have occurred otherwise.

Route of Administration. All medical specialists must convince certain patients to follow long-term or life-long medication, but psychiatrists face an especially difficult problem. When chronic patients relapse, they often become withdrawn, hostile and uncooperative. At this time, when they may benefit most, they usually stop taking their medicine. Coping with this requires the cooperation of the patient's family and the services of a visiting nurse, often over an extended time period. When failure occurs, administer intramuscular injections of a long-acting phenothiazine in an oil (prolixin decanoate) base every two to three weeks.

PHARMACEUTICAL PREPARATIONS

The most effective way of taking oral phenothiazines is by liquid oral ingestion. This is the quickest method and provides more complete absorption, then the whole tablet; the spansule is the least effective. Since phenothiazines are excreted slowly, there is no advantage for the spansule.

Intramuscular dosage is calculated at half the oral dose, but confirmatory data are lacking. Sometimes, although it is rare, severe orthostatic hypotension can occur. Consequently, a test may be tried first while monitoring the patient's blood pressure. In emergencies, this test may have to be omitted. For this reason, many physicians use high-potency drugs such as thiothixene, haloperidol, perphenazine, fluphenazine, or trifluoperazine for intramuscular administration since they have a much lower prevalence of postural hypotension.

Fluphenazine enanthate or fluphenazine decanoate in oil form is injected deep into the muscle for long-term intramuscular treatment. Due to its slow, even absorption, it produces an effect lasting from one to three weeks. This is desirable in patients who cannot be trusted to take their drugs. The IM dose is usually between 25 and 100 mg; although many psychiatrists start the patient right off at home on this medication, you should, when possible, stabilize the patient on fluphenazine tablets, and then switch to the injectable form. In this way, side effects are minimized, but when this is impractical, go directly to the intramuscular administration. The reason we recommend this is that a day-to-day treatment allows a more convenient mechanism for arriving at the proper clinical adjustment of dosage. After this, we switch to the depot form. The differences between methods of administration are minor; however, empirical results have shown that depot intramuscular medication can be used from the beginning, even with acutely decompensated schizophrenic patients, and the differences between oral and depot are marginal.

Although 25 mg of the enanthate or decanoate every two weeks has been widely used, flexibility of a starting dose and intervals between does prevent side effects and improves clinical results. Intramuscular therapy should be initiated with a low dose to prevent adverse reactions, and maintenance should be achieved with the least amount given as infrequently as possible. The periods of maximum risk for the various EPS after depot fluphenazine are as follows: dystonia, 12–24 hours after injection; akathisia, 1–4 days after injection; and parkinsonism, 2–5 days after injection. Of course, extrapyramidal side effects can occur at any time point; thus, for this time course one should remain particularly alert.

Controlled studies comparing fluphenazine decanoate and enanthate indicate that they are nearly equal in all their properties except that the decanoate is slightly longer acting and produces slightly fewer side effects. Most controlled studies show the decanoate or enanthate form equal to the oral. A few studies show the long-acting intramuscular form to be superior for maintenance, probably because of poor compliance in the group receiving oral medication.

CAUTIONS WHEN PRESCRIBING PHENOTHIAZINES

This section includes a partial listing of cautions; see also sections on elderly patients (below) and side effects (p. 61). When drugs are given in high doses, and particularly if they are given intramuscularly, patients should be cautioned against postural hypotension.

Previous history of cardiovascular or liver disease provides a caution, but not a contraindication.

Excessive sun exposure—Severe phototoxic skin burns can occur with chlorpromazine and other phenothiazines in a few hours under the summer sun. Patients must be warned of this danger and advised to use protective clothing or a spray that blocks ultraviolet rays.

Elderly Patients

These patients tolerate reduced dosages of phenothiazines and are more likely to suffer the following side effects.

- *Cardiovascular effects*—Orthostatic hypotension can be annoying and, in rare instances, quite dangerous in older patients. Since cardiovascular disease is common in the elderly, they may have less of a tolerance for hypotension.
- *Agranulocytosis* occurs with greater frequency in the elderly female.
- *Prostate and bladder difficulties* are more of a problem, as is constipation caused by phenothiazine treatment.
- *Glaucoma*—Only the narrow angle type can be worsened, but you must guard against this because damage to eyesight can result.
- *Depression or delirium*—Some old people suffer depression or delirium from excess phenothiazine dosage.

ANTIPSYCHOTIC EFFECTIVENESS

Pierre Deniker noted, in describing his and Jean Delay's initial experiment with chlorpromazine in 1952, "We had scarcely treated 10 patients—with all due respect to the fervent adherents of statistics—when our conviction proved correct." Now, more than 25 years later, no doubt exists, clinical or statistical, that chlorpromazine is significantly more effective for acute schizophrenics than placebos or sedatives (Table 3.3). Double-blind studies establish this unequivocally.

The drug-placebo difference can be quantified by looking at the

Table 3.3
Chlorpromazine-Placebo Comparisons at Different Levels

Dose (mg/day)	No. of studies in which chlorpromazine was		
	More effective than placebo	Slightly more effective than placebo	Equal to placebo
300 or less	11	6	9
301–400	4	3	1
401–500	4	0	1
501–800	14	0	0
>800	12	0	0
Totals (all doses)	15	9	11

percentage of patients who recover or very much improve vs. the percentage of patients who become worse on placebo and on drug. These data, plus that on patients who show no change or minimal improvement, are shown in Figure 3.5A. A substantial drug-placebo difference can be seen, with approximately three times as many patients doing better on drug than on placebo. Most importantly, however, a very large percentage of patients deteriorate on placebo in comparison to those who deteriorate on drugs. It is impossible to make any quantitative comparison between the drugs for one disease and different drugs for another disease. However, quantification of the drug-placebo difference allows a qualitative comparison.

A double-blind study by the British Medical Research Council with random assignment of streptomycin plus bed rest, in comparison to just bed rest, provides a convenient example. Streptomycin plus bed rest was substantially better than just bed rest alone.

The classic antibiotics are penicillin for pneumococcal pneumonia and streptomycin for tuberculosis. No placebo data exist for pneumococcal pneumonia since the sulfa drugs were standard treatment for pneumonia when penicillin was discovered. The death rate from pneumococcal pneumonia with sulfonamides was 11.8%. This dropped to 6.3% when penicillin was used to treat pneumococcal pneumonia.

We caution against any but a qualitative comparison since the seriousness of the disease, its natural history, and the drug-placebo difference need to be considered. Note that the quantitative mag-

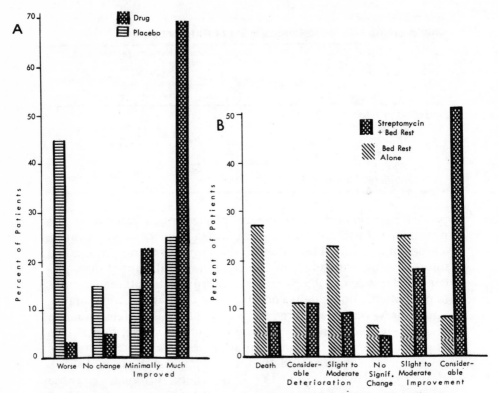

Figure 3.5. *A*, result of treatment of schizophrenic patients with antipsychotic drugs or placebo. *B*, therapeutic effects of streptomycin with bed rest vs. bed rest alone in pulmonary tuberculosis.

nitude of the drug-placebo difference is substantial with all three medications.

We have addressed ourselves to the drug-placebo difference for acute patients. A related, but different, question is whether failure to treat with antipsychotic drugs for an extended period of time can result in permanent harm to the patient. May and Toma did a particularly important study in terms of this specific issue. Patients were randomly assigned to drugs or no drugs and they were also randomly assigned to receive psychotherapy or no psychotherapy. Parenthetically, we should add that the psychotherapy was two sessions/week which was administered by residents, and probably does not clearly constitute an adequate trial. Most importantly, however, was the comparison of drug and no drug. The essential methodological variable in this study was length of treatment. The experimental design called for 6 months to 1 year of treatment either without drugs or with drugs. Most controlled studies last only 4 to 6 weeks. Thus, a study lasting 6 months to 1 year is quite unique. Patients who received drugs did substantially better on a number of variables than patients who did not receive drugs. However, essentially all patients had some degree of recovery from their illness. In part, this can be attributed to the passage of time and the fact that patients who failed on no drug could receive drugs after 6 months to 1 year. Note that these patients were first admission schizophrenics. After the study ended, all patients could receive all indicated psychiatric treatments. The patients were then followed for the next 3 to 5 years. Both treatments were clinical and, in that sense, similar during this time period. Considering the similarity in treatment, we can now determine perhaps whether there are any long-term effects from having drug or no drug initially for an extended period of time. More specifically, would the failure to treat with drugs result in permanent harm to the patient? As an index of how well the patients were doing, the authors calculated the number of days in the hospital during this time period (Fig. 3.6). They roughly equated many brief hospitalizations against a few long hospitalizations. Note: the patients who initially received drugs did much better during the follow-up than those who did not receive drugs initially. This indicates that living through a lengthy hospitalization without medication, results in some sort of permanent harm. The mechanism for this is not yet known. It may be that the dopamine blockade of the antipsychotics in some sense reduces some biological aspects of the psychotic process; i.e., the disease does not progress as much with medication. An alternative explanation could be that long hospitalization severs social ties which are important to a patient's continuous functioning. These social supports are lost due to the long hospitalization and they may not be regained. Whatever the mechanism, there is a substantial difference in the long-term follow-up of patients treated with drugs or without drugs. It thus appears that drugs alter the natural history of schizophrenia.

CHOOSING ANTIPSYCHOTICS

Many phenothiazine drugs plus four other classes of antipsychotics are available on the American market. Like digitalis prep-

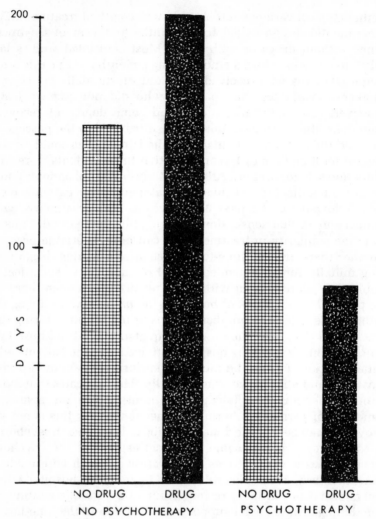

Figure 3.6. Three years' follow-up after first release.

arations, they are more alike than different. Criteria for choosing one antipsychotic over another include the following considerations.

Side Effects

The difference in side effects among the antipsychotics is much greater than their difference in clinical effects. A drug that produces much drowsiness may be preferable for a patient with insomnia, whereas one that produces little or none is preferred for an outpatient; the improvement rate of both is about equal.

Knowledge

Familiarize yourself with several antipsychotics with different properties.

Cost

Since you may have to use high doses for extended time periods, cost is important to both hospital and patient. You can easily see the differences in price by calculating equivalency (see Tables 3.4 and 3.5 for cost estimates). The cost of the various antipsychotic agents is roughly comparable, differing only by a factor of about two. This might mean a difference of $0.25 per day—insignificant when weighed against the need to avoid an unwanted side effect in a particular patient.

Drug History

If an agent previously produced good results for the patient, use it again. If a drug failed or caused a significant side effect, use another. Although differences in clinical efficiency are virtually impossible to distinguish in large samples, many reports exist demonstrating that a patient showing no response to one preparation improves dramatically when given another. The following is a schema of different phenothiazine classes.

Differences Among Aliphatics, Piperazines and Piperidines

Therapeutic effects are the same. In actuality, differences lie in the side effects characteristically produced by the three phenothiazine groups (Scheme 1).

Aliphatics

This group produces more
- Sedation
- Hypotension
- Dermatitis
- Convulsions
- Atropine-like side effects
- Agranulocytosis

but fewer extrapyramidal side effects (EPS) than do piperazines.

Table 3.4

Patient Cost for Antipsychotic Medication

Drug	Doses used in controlled study		Total daily dose	$ per patient 30 days—average dose	Experts dose range	Experts dose ratio
	Dose ratio	SEM				
Chlorpromazine (Thorazine)	100		734	10.73	15–1500	100
Triflupromazine (Vesprin)	28.4 ± 1.8		208	46.90	75–400	28
Thioridazine (Mellaril)	95.3 ± 8.2		700	31.45	150–800	100
Prochlorperazine (Compazine)	14.3 ± 1.7		105	23.99	25–150	15
Perphenazine (Trilafon)	8.9 ± .6		65.1	26.75	12–60	10.0
Fluphenazine (Prolixin)	1.2 ± .1		8.8	10.48	3–45	1.8
Fluphenazine (Prolixin decanoate)	.67		4.9	21.44	—	—
Trifluoperazine (Stelazine)	2.8 ± .4		20.6	13.04	10–40	5
Acetophenazine (Tindal)	23.5 ± 1.5		172	22.24	40–160	18.7
Carphenazine (Proketazine)	24.3 ± 2.7		176	19.65	60–400	28
Butaperazine (Repoise)	8.9 ± 1.1		65	15.99	25–110	13.7
Mesoridazine (Serentil)	55.3 ± 8.3		406	25.83	75–400	55
Piperacetazine (Quide)	10.5		77.1	39.12	20–160	6.0
Haloperidol (Haldol)	1.6 ± .4		11.4	14.45	2–16	2.5
Chlorprothixene (Taractan)	43.9 ± 13.9		322	25.83	40–600	100
Thiothixene (Navane)	5.2 ± 1.8		38	25.61	10–60	4.8
Molindone (Moban)	6.0		44	12.13	—	10
Loxapine (Loxitane)	8.7		64	14.80	—	—

Because of their high initial sedative capability, aliphatics have been favored by some for treating excited, assaultive, hospitalized schizophrenics. High-dose oral chlorpromazine (Thorazine), in particular, has been used. Actually, any phenothiazine can theo-

Table 3.5
Cost per Milligram for Different Tablet Size

Drug	Percentage of cost at most inexpensive tablet size													
	200	100	50	25	16	125	10	8	5	4	25	2	1	0.5
Chlorpromazine	100	180	300	500			1060							
Triflupromazine			100	150			250							
Thioridazine	100	138	231	415			762							
Prochlorperazine				100			210		323					
Perphenazine					100			149		246		358		
Fluphenazine									100		154		270	
Trifluoperazine							100		153			353	553	
Carphenazine		100	165		277									
Butaperazine				100			197		310					
Mesoridazine		100	167	289			545							
Piperacetazine				100			167							
Haloperidol									100					
Chlorprothixene		100	165	271			494					178	238	332
Thiothixene							100		151				291	450

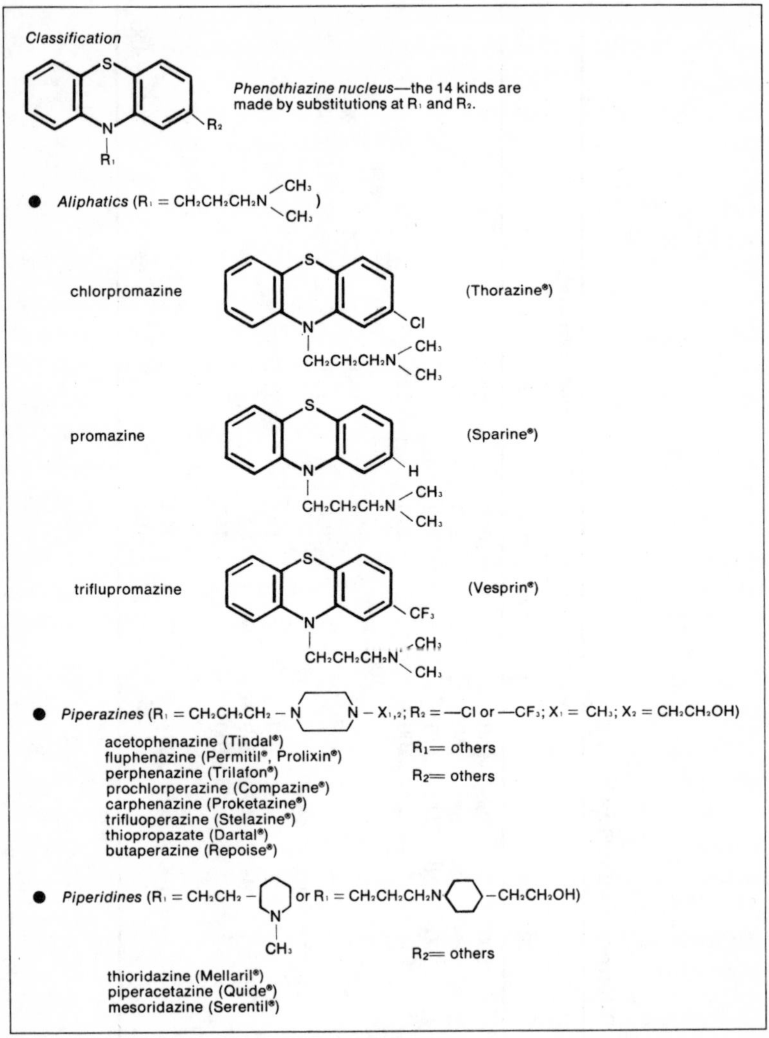

Classification

Phenothiazine nucleus—the 14 kinds are made by substitutions at R_1 and R_2.

● *Aliphatics* ($R_1 = CH_2CH_2CH_2N \begin{smallmatrix} CH_3 \\ CH_3 \end{smallmatrix}$)

chlorpromazine — Cl — $CH_2CH_2CH_2N \begin{smallmatrix} CH_3 \\ CH_3 \end{smallmatrix}$ — (Thorazine®)

promazine — H — $CH_2CH_2CH_2N \begin{smallmatrix} CH_3 \\ CH_3 \end{smallmatrix}$ — (Sparine®)

triflupromazine — CF_3 — $CH_2CH_2CH_2N \begin{smallmatrix} CH_3 \\ CH_3 \end{smallmatrix}$ — (Vesprin®)

● *Piperazines* ($R_1 = CH_2CH_2CH_2 - N \underset{}{\bigcirc} N - X_{1,2}$; $R_2 = -Cl$ or $-CF_3$; $X_1 = CH_3$; $X_2 = CH_2CH_2OH$)

acetophenazine (Tindal®)
fluphenazine (Permitil®, Prolixin®) R_1= others
perphenazine (Trilafon®)
prochlorperazine (Compazine®) R_2= others
carphenazine (Proketazine®)
trifluoperazine (Stelazine®)
thiopropazate (Dartal®)
butaperazine (Repoise®)

● *Piperidines* ($R_1 = CH_2CH_2 - \underset{\underset{CH_3}{|}}{\bigcirc}$ or $R_1 = CH_2CH_2CH_2N\langle\rangle-CH_2CH_2OH$)

        R_2= others

thioridazine (Mellaril®)
piperacetazine (Quide®)
mesoridazine (Serentil®)

Scheme 1

retically be used in massive doses until either a therapeutic result or a serious side effect is produced. The French, for example, use trifluoperazine (Stelazine) in 700-mg daily doses. The long experience using chlorpromazine when massive oral doses are required has fostered confidence, but the custom has been changing to the use of piperazines, thiothixene, loxapine and haloperidol in intra-muscular treatment because chlorpromazine produces pain at the injection site, as well as excessive sedation and postural hypoten-sion. Yet no studies clearly demonstrate that the higher sedative capacity of massive-dose chlorpromazine is preferable to equiva-lent doses of a piperazine, such as perphenazine (Trilafon), trifluo-perazine (Stelazine) or fluphenazine (Prolixin) in acutely excited schizophrenics.

Chlorpromazine sedation produces both an undesirable side effect and a necessary clinical effect. The desired result is to calm an excited or assaultive patient. Fifty percent of the schizophrenics taking chlorpromazine become drowsy or fatigued during the first 10 therapy days, whereas only 20% of those on trifluoperazine do so. This does not necessarily mean that 2000 mg of chlorprom-azine calm an assaultive patient more effectively than do 100 mg of trifluoperazine.

In addition, outpatients who must be alert may be very disturbed by the initial chlorpromazine sedation. They feel much more comfortable with perphenazine, fluphenazine (Permitil, Prolixin) or trifluoperazine. Chlorpromazine causes fewer extrapyramidal side effects (EPS) than the piperazine derivatives.

Piperazines

This group produces more EPS and less sedation, hypotension and lens opacities. These drugs are preferred when there is a need to avoid sedation, for example, for college students taking exams, for older patients prone to postural hypotension, or for hyperten-sives in whom a large blood pressure drop would endanger coro-nary or cerebral blood flow.

Extrapyramidal side effects, on the other hand, can be annoying and frightening.

Piperidines

Thioridazine (Mellaril), the prototype of this group, produces *more* electrocardiogram disturbance, retinal toxicity, ejaculatory inhibition and *fewer* EPS. Thioridazine is widely used in the United States, having earned its reputation with its low EPS incidence. Its usefulness is limited by the incidence of pigmentary retinopathy, reported only in doses over 1200 mg. A dosage ceiling of 800 mg daily has now been placed on the package insert. This is the only warranted and rational upper daily dosage limit of an antipsychotic drug.

The 800-mg thioridazine ceiling limits its usefulness for acutely hospitalized schizophrenics, as does the lack of an injectable form. Nevertheless, the lower EPS incidence makes thioridazine a desirable drug.

Ejaculation inhibition may be disturbing to young males who are able to achieve erection but are unable to ejaculate. This side effect has been used with therapeutic success in men suffering from premature ejaculation.

Thioridazine produces flattening of the T wave and an increased QR interval. This effect may be caused by a benign repolarization disturbance that disappears when the drug is withdrawn. Our present knowledge indicates these EKG changes are without clinical significance. Severe cardiac arrhythmias and sudden death have been attributed to piperadine phenothiazines, but it is unlikely that these drugs were causally responsible.

In trying to glean the best qualities of thioridazine while eliminating the worst, piperacetazine (Quide) and mesoridazine (Serentil) have recently been introduced.

Mesoridazine is more effective for treating acute and chronic schizophrenia than is placebo (Table 3.6) and is equivalent to chlorpromazine (Tables 3.7 and 3.8). Piperacetazine and mesoridazine have the same type of side effects as do the other antipsychotic drugs. Electrocardiographic alterations resembling those caused by quinidine and hypokalemia may occur with mesoridazine. All effects are reversible by reducing the dose or stopping the drug. No ocular changes (e.g., pigmentary retinopathy) have been associated with mesoridazine to date, but possibly they may occur. Mesoridazine is available in both oral and intramuscular forms.

Piperacetazine's effectiveness as compared with phenothiazines has not been established, but several controlled studies suggest it is equal to the others (Tables 3.7 and 3.8). No advantages have been demonstrated over related compounds with respect to clinical effectiveness or adverse reactions. Piperacetazine is available in oral form only.

Butyrophenones

General Description

The butyrophenones have antipsychotic effects equal to the

Table 3.6

Drug-Placebo Comparisons in Double-Blind Controlled Studies of Schizophrenia

Drug	Number of Studies	Percentage of studies in which drug was	
		More effective than placebo	Equal to placebo
Phenothiazines			
Chlorpromazine	66	83.00	17
Trifluoperazine	18	88.9	11.1
Triflupromazine	10	90.0	10.0
Thioridazine	7	100.0	0.0
Mesoridazine	3	100.0	0
Perphenazine	5	100.0	0.0
Butaperazine	4	100.0	0.0
Prochlorperazine	9	77.8	22.2
Fluphenazine	15	100.0	0
Carphenazine	2	100.0	0
Mepazine	5	40	60
Promazine	7	43	57
Others			
Reserpine	29	69.0	31.0
Phenobarbital	3	0.0	100.0
Chlorprothixene	4	100.0	0.0
Thiothixene	2	100.0	0.0
Haloperidol	9	100.0	0.0
Molindone (Moban)	1	100	
Loxapine (Loxitane)	6	83.3	16.7

phenothiazines. Haloperidol (Haldol) is the only one available in this country for psychiatric use and is ·one of the more commonly prescribed antipsychotic agents in America.

Like the phenothiazines and thioxanthenes, the butyrophenones have a three-carbon straight chain attached to a nitrogen.

Chlorine replacement in haloperidol by other halogens produces methylperidol, bromoperidol, trifluperisol and clofluperidol. Replacing the phenyl nucleus altogether has produced dipiperon, droperidol, benzperidol, haloanisone and spiroperidol. Two more recently synthesized compounds are the long-acting pimozide and fluspirilene, although technically they are no longer butyrophenones.

Replacing the phenyl nucleus greatly alters potency and duration of action of butyrophenones. Droperidol (Inapsine) thus has a rapid onset, a short duration, a potent antipsychotic and an

Table 3.7

Comparisons of Phenothiazines with Chlorpromazine in Double-Blind Controlled Studies of Schizophrenia

Drug	Number of studies	Percentage of studies in which		
		Drug was more effective than chlorpromazine	Drug was equal to chlorpromazine	Drug was less effective than chlorpromazine
Trifluoperazine	11	0.0	100.0	0.0
Butaperazine	2	0.0	100	0
Triflupromazine	10	0.0	100.0	0.0
Thioridazine	12	0.0	100.0	0.0
Mesoridazine	7	0	100	0
Perphenazine	6	0.0	100.0	0.0
Carphenazine	2	0	100.0	0
Prochlorperazine	10	0.0	100.0	0.0
Acetophenazine	1	0	100.0	0.0
Fluphenazine	9	0.0	100.0	0.0
Thiopropazate	1	0	100	0
Mepazine	4	0.0	0.0	100.0
Piperacetazine	3	0	100.0	0
Promazine	6	0.0	33.3	66.7
Chlorprothixine	6	0	100	0
Thiothixene	4	0	100	0
Haloperidol	3	0	100	0
Phenobarbital	6	0	100	0
Molindone	6	0	100	0
Loxapine	15	0	93	7

antiemetic effect. This drug is used in the United States only as an adjunct to anesthesia, but also has potential in psychiatric emergencies.

Haloperidol (Haldol)

Clinical Use and Effectiveness

Haloperidol is rapidly absorbed from the gastrointestinal tract, reaching its highest plasma level in 2 to 5 hours, and is slowly excreted. High doses have been found to be safe. At present, 100 mg/day is the maximal dose according to the *Physicians' Desk Reference*.

Injectable haloperidol is frequently used in emergency room treatment for violent psychotics. In fact, intramuscular haloperidol administered 5 mg hourly is a widely used regimen for such

Table 3.8
Comparison of Antipsychotic Agents to Thioridazine and Trifluoperazine as Standard Phenothiazines*

	No. of studies	Percentage of studies		
		More effective than thioridazine	Equal to thioridazine	Less effective
Mesoridazine	2	0	100	0
Carphenazine	1	0	100	0
Piperacetazine	3	0	100	0
Haloperidol	2	0	100	0
		More effective than trifluoperazine	Equal to trifluoperazine	Less effective
Mesoridazine	1	0	100	0
Carphenazine	3	0	100	0
Acetophenazine	1	0	100	0
Butaperazine	3	0	100	0
Chlorprothixene	1	0	100	0
Haloperidol	4	0	100	0

* Studies placed are in this table only if chlorpromazine was not used, so that this information is based upon different studies than that in Table 2.3.

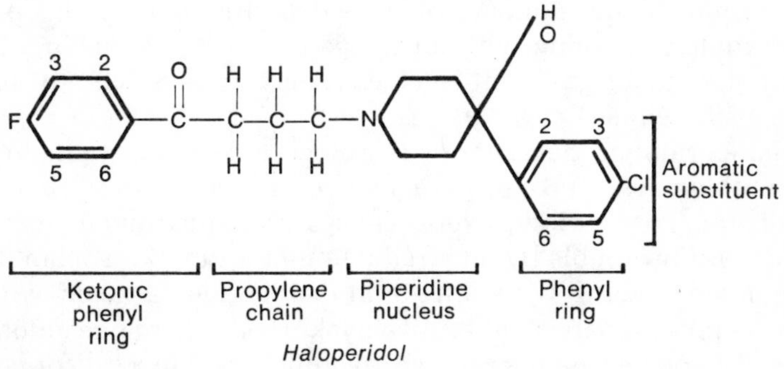
H
O
3 2
F
5 6
O
H H H
C C C C N
H H H
2 3
Cl
6 5
Aromatic substituent
Ketonic phenyl ring
Propylene chain
Piperidine nucleus
Phenyl ring
Haloperidol

Scheme 2

patients. Minimal undesirable sedation and hypotension occur, at least with the fairly low doses used so far.

A colorless, odorless, tasteless liquid form exists. While similar to chlorpromazine in antimanic activity, haloperidol is not clearly superior. Only in the Gilles de la Tourette syndrome does primacy seem established, although definitive data are lacking.

Pharmacologic and Side Effects

The side effects of haloperidol are mainly EPS. Butyrophenones cause little hypotension, hypothermia or other autonomic nervous system changes and have only weak anticholinergic properties.

Butyrophenones do not adversely interact with oral antidiabetic agents, anticonvulsants, digitalis, other cardiovascular drugs or diuretics. Therefore, many regard them as one of the drugs of choice for psychotic patients with cardiac disease.

Because they are not potentiated by alcohol, patients can drink in moderation two weeks after beginning haloperidol treatment.

Haloperidol causes fewer autonomic side effects, sedation and dizziness than does chlorpromazine. Using haloperidol in the elderly or in patients with cardiovascular disease appears rational, although piperazine phenothiazines are equally safe.

In rare instances, the so-called "malignant syndrome" causes dehydrating hyperthermia and a clouded state. This syndrome occurred long before antipsychotic drugs were discovered and probably is falsely attributed to haloperidol It has been called "lethal catatonia," and since it occurred before drugs were discovered, it is probably a variant of schizophrenia. Adequate administration of fluids is important since dehydration may be a part of the problem. Cooling with an ice pack can be life saving. If the fever rises to a significant level, electroconvulsive therapy should be considered (see page 70).

Haloperidol produces more neurologic side effects than do most phenothiazines. EPS are perhaps even more common than with chlorpromazine. Haloperidol causes extrapyramidal reactions which are reversible by dose reduction or antiparkinsonian drugs. The main hazard with long-term haloperidol use, as with all neuroleptics, is persistent tardive dyskinesia. Allergic reactions are rare. No ocular damage, liver dysfunction, blood disorders or phototoxicity have been proven to be causally related to haloperidol.

Thioxanthenes

The thioxanthenes differ from the phenothiazines by substitution of a carbon with a double bond for the nitrogen in the number

10 position of the central ring. Controlled and uncontrolled studies since 1959 show that thioxanthenes possess clinical effects similar to those of the phenothiazines.

Chlorprothixene (Taractan)

The thioxanthene analog of chlorpromazine, chlorprothixene produces side effects, similar to those of chlorpromazine.

Thiothixene (Navane)

Navane is a high-extrapyramidal, low-sedation antipsychotic drug similar to fluphenazine or haloperidol in its properties. It is minimally sedating and may actually be activating at low doses. It has been clearly shown to produce antipsychotic effects equal to those of the other antipsychotics. Lenticular opacities are reported in rare instances after prolonged use. (See discussion of chlorpromazine-produced lenticular opacities, page 71.)

Indoles and Dibenzoxapines

Two new agents, molindone (which has an indole structure) and loxapine (which belongs to the dibenzoxapine category), have clearly been shown to have antipsychotic effects (Table 3.9). Six controlled studies involving approximately 200 patients found molindone similar in efficacy to the standard antipsychotic drug:

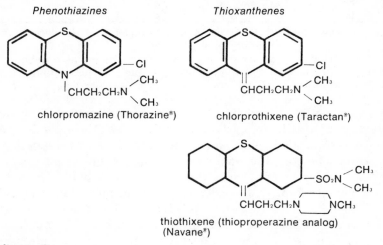

Phenothiazines

chlorpromazine (Thorazine®)

Thioxanthenes

chlorprothixene (Taractan®)

thiothixene (thioproperazine analog)
(Navane®)

Scheme 3

Table 3.9

Summary of Studies on the Antipsychotic Efficacy of Loxapine and Molindone in Schizophrenia

Investigators	No. of patients	Patient group (schizo-phrenics)	Outcome*
Clark et al. (1975)	37	Newly admitted	lox = tri > pla†
Denber (1970)	31	Newly admitted	lox = tri
Moore (1975)	57	Newly admitted	lox > CPZ
Shopsin et al. (1972)	30	Newly admitted	lox < CPZ
Simpson and Cuculic (1976)	43	Newly admitted	lox = tri
Smith (pers. comm.)	12	Newly admitted	lox = tri
Steinbook et al. (1973)	54	Newly admitted	lox = CPZ‡
Van Der Velde and Kilte (1975)	25	Newly admitted	lox = thi > pla
Charalampous et al. (1974)	54	Subacute	lox = pla < thi
Bishop and Gallant (1970)	24	Chronic	lox = tri
Clark et al. (1972)	50	Chronic	lox = CPZ > pla
Moyano (1975)	48	Chronic	lox = tri
Schiele (1975)	49	Chronic	lox = CPZ
Simpson et al. (1971)	52	Acute	mol = tri
Clark et al. (1970)	43	Chronic	mol = CPZ > pla
Freeman and Frederick (1969)	28	Chronic	mol = tri
Gallant and Bishop (1968)	43	Chronic	mol = tri
Ramsey et al. (1970)	20	Chronic	mol = tri

* Abbreviations: lox, loxapine; mol, molindone; tri, trifluoperazine; thi, thiothixene; CPZ, chlorpromazine; pla, placebo.

† Use of equals sign means any overall difference which might exist could not be detected on basis of number of patients, population, etc.

‡ lox > CPZ on some, but not all measures.

it was slightly superior in one study, not different in three and slightly inferior in two. Clark and associates (1970) conducted a placebo-controlled study and found molindone to be superior to placebo. Qualitatively, molindone improves the same range of schizophrenic symptoms as the other antipsychotic agents and had similar prophylactic effects. Although molindone generally produces the same range of extrapyramidal and autonomic side effects as the phenothiazines, it differs in that it does not induce weight gain. Also, since it does not inhibit the noradrenaline (norepinephrine) uptake pump mechanism, it probably does not interfere with the hypotensive action of guanethidine.

Clark and associates (1972, 1975) have provided the best evidence on the efficacy of loxapine. They tested loxapine in carefully executed double-blind studies in hospitalized patients with chronic and acute schizophrenia. In all three studies, loxapine was significantly superior to placebo. Van Der Velde and Kiltie (1975) also found loxapine superior to placebo. In another 15 studies involving about 600 patients, loxapine was found to be indistinguishable from standard antipsychotics in 12 of those studies and superior in one study. In contrast, another study found loxapine more effective than thiothixene in younger, but not in older, patients, while one group found loxapine less effective than thiothixene and another found loxapine less effective than chlorpromazine. Considered as a group it seems that loxapine is an effective antipsychotic. It has the same range of side effects as the other antipsychotics. Both new antipsychotics are effective drugs and their use is recommended. No occular, liver, blood, or phototoxicity has been reported.

Rauwolfia alkaloids

The phenothiazines, butyrophenones and thioxanthenes are clearly more effective antipsychotics than are the rauwolfia alkaloids.

The rauwolfia alkaloids decrease storage of catecholamines but do not alter membrane uptake. They are, at present, rarely used for their antipsychotic properties. They do produce extrapyramidal side effects. These drugs have been used experimentally to treat tardive dyskinesia.

Side effects are primarily those of parasympathetic predominance (excessive salivation, nasal congestion, excessive gastric secretion), nausea, diarrhea, orthostatic hypotension, bradycardia and cutaneous vasodilation.

An occasional case of mental depression is encountered in hypertensives treated with rauwolfia alkaloids. This can, at times, be severe.

CHOICE OF ANTIPSYCHOTICS

In one National Institute of Mental Health study, chlorpromazine was found superior to fluphenazine in apathetic and retarded schizophrenics. Note: this contradicts the widely held view that piperazines (especially Stelazine) should be used in withdrawn patients. This finding was not replicated in a subsequent study. Although tentative findings have suggested that certain subtype patients seem to respond better to certain drugs, further research to match a specific antipsychotic agent with a particular patient has failed to confirm these initial findings. All antipsychotics are equally effective in all subtypes.

All Phenothiazines Have Been Found Equally Effective for Treating Schizophrenia

Exceptions are mepazine (withdrawn from the market) and promazine (Sparine). No phenothiazine combination is more effective than chlorpromazine alone (see Tables 2.3 and 2.4).

Other Clinical Uses of Antipsychotics

- *Manic reactions*—Antipsychotics can be used alone or in combination with lithium.
- *Symptomatic psychoses*—The primary cause must, of course, also be eliminated. Antipsychotic drugs are useful for symptomatic treatment.
- *Amphetamine psychosis*—Antipsychotics are the drugs of choice in psychoses *known* to be produced by psychomotor stimulants such as amphetamines or methylphenidate.
- *Induced psychoses*—A firm guideline cannot be set since many street-sold drugs are impure, having a dubious pharmacology: i.e., the patient may not know what is being ingested. Because antipsychotics exhibit atropine-like side effects themselves, they are contraindicated in atropine psychosis (the central anticholinergic syndrome). They may even exacerbate this syndrome. It may not be advisable to use pharmacological agents, but rather to talk the patient down, since what the patient actually ingested is unknown.
- *Psychotic children*—Can be effectively drug-treated.
- *Agitated depression*—Phenothiazines are sometimes as effective as tricyclics. In retarded depressions, tricyclics retain the edge. In depression, phenothiazines have the advantage of lower lethal potential in the event of overdose, but the disadvantage of tardive dyskinesia.
- *Intractable hiccough*—Is treatable.
- *Chronic brain syndromes*—Can be symptomatically treated.

SIDE EFFECTS

Adverse Behavioral Effects

Drowsiness

A common symptom during the first few days of treatment, drowsiness usually disappears in one or two weeks. Chlorpromazine and thioridazine produces more sedation (about 80% of patients) than the piperazine phenothiazines.

Rare Effects

- Depression—Unlike the rauwolfia alkaloids, phenothiazines rarely cause depression. When melancholia occurs in a phenothiazine patient, an affective manifestation of an extrapyramidal reaction should be ruled out (see below under "akinesia").
- Feelings of unreality.

Withdrawal Symptoms

The antipsychotics do not cause withdrawal symptoms of the barbiturate or narcotic type, and are in no sense addicting. Patients never tend to abuse these drugs by self medicating with higher doses. Their withdrawal does not produce convulsions or any other manifestations of the barbiturate withdrawal syndrome, nor does it produce narcotic withdrawal symptoms.

With the sudden cessation of high-dose phenothiazine, the patient may experience gastrointestinal symptoms (nausea, vomiting, diarrhea).

It has been suggested that these symptoms may arise from the withdrawal of the antiparkinsonian medications.

Toxic Effects on the Central Nervous System

Extrapyramidal Side Effects (EPS)

These occur in about 15 to 30% of patients treated with phenothiazines and are more likely to be caused by piperazines than by aliphatics.

- Pseudoparkinsonism—This constitutes about 40% of all EPS and is composed most often of: akinesia, muscle rigidity, tremor, changes in posture, drooling, mask-like facies, shuffling gait and loss of associated movements.

The most likely pathophysiology is through blockage of dopamine receptors in basal ganglia by the antipsychotic.

- *Akathisia* derives from Greek and means the "inability to sit"; it is a syndrome in which the patient cannot remain still. He constantly paces, often making chewing and lip movements, finger and leg movements. The patient is driven and cannot concentrate. He may try to rationalize night-time agitation by saying that he awoke because of bad dreams or the need to urinate. Patients often erroneously attribute their painful agitation to a psychological source.

Helpful Distinguishing Characteristics for Akathisia

Akathisia	*Anxiety, agitation, psychotic relapse*
Driven by motor restlessness and unable to concentrate on voicing symptoms	Can concentrate on expressing symptoms at length
Symptoms primarily motor and cannot be controlled by the patient's will	Symptoms controllable
Worsened by dosage increase	Relieved by dosage increase
Can be relieved by reduction of offending drug	Symptoms worsened by lowering dosage
At times only responsiveness to antiparkinsonian agents distinguishes from anxiety or increased psychotic agitation	Unresponsive to antiparkinsonian agents

---

The physician must rely on his observation of motor restlessness and pacing to detect akathisia. If you too readily accept a psychodynamic explanation, you can miss this condition.

When misdiagnosed as anxiety, tension or psychiatric exacerbation, the physician usually prescribes more antipsychotic which worsens the akathisia. Correct recognition leads to treatment with an antiparkinsonian drug and not to more antipsychotic. The differential diagnosis can be difficult, and this common side effect is missed too often (50% of all EPS). If anticholinergics fail to resolve the akathesia, one may try benzodiazepines.

- *Dystonias*—These dramatically alarming EPS usually occur within the first five days, sometimes in as little as an hour, and almost never after the first three months of oral phenothiazine treatment. (They can occur after each injection of depot medication.)

    Dystonias include spasms of eye, neck, back or other muscles (oculogyric crisis, torticollis, opisthotonos).

    This side effect must be distinguished from hysteria, catatonia, and tetanus. Before they were widely recognized, dyskinesias were misdiagnosed as tetany, meningitis, encephalitis, hysteria, acute psychosis and malingering.

    Akinesia is an EPS in which there is a decrease in spontaneity, gestures, and speech. The patient is apathetic and can be confused with one who is depressed, demoralized, or is a residual schizophrenic.

- *Persistent (tardive) dyskinesia*—This syndrome usually starts late in the course of long-term antipsychotic administration. It consists of gross hyperkinetic activity in the oral region (lip smacking and sucking, jaw movements, "fly-catcher" tongue movement). Choreiform-like and even athetoid movements of the extremities of the body also occur. Swallowing may become a problem with resulting weight loss. In an unknown percentage of cases the syndrome is apparently irreversible. The movements disappear during sleep.

Tardive dyskinesia (TD) is usually found in elderly chronic schizophrenics. It is slightly more prevalent in elderly women who have complicated drug, somatic therapy (electroconvulsive therapy, leukotomy), organic brain syndrome and ingestion (alcohol, dietary, poisons) histories. The relationship of sex may be an artifact of age since women live longer than men. Young patients on phenothiazine for only three to six months sometimes, but rarely, get it. Although many cases are irreversible, many patients recover completely when antipsychotic drugs are discontinued. After discontinuance the tardive dyskinesia symptoms generally worsen in the first weeks, and then gradually improve until they disappear completely in a significant number of cases. Unfortunately, the antipsychotic drugs may suppress tardive dyskinesia symptoms even though they are causing the damage which produced this syndrome. In essence, then, the drug masks its own side effects. If a patient shows even questionable symptomatology, it is important to discontinue antipsychotic treatment immediately. Patients generally do not relapse immediately upon discontinuance of antipsychotics, so in many instances a trial period off antipsychotics does not produce deterioration of the psychiatric condition. The worsening of symptoms provides evidence that it is indeed tardive dyskinesia, and this confirms the diagnosis. If this is the case, patients should be managed off neuroleptics completely, if possible. Of course, in many cases antipsychotics are necessary to treat the schizophrenic illness so that the clinician must prescribe antipsychotics, but the knowledge that tardive dyskinesia is developing is important, so that the clinician can be particularly careful in using minimal amounts of antipsychotics.

TD may be the most common serious unwanted result of antipsychotic drug use, with reported prevalence in chronically hospitalized psychiatric patients from 2% to over 50%. It is believed to be caused by the functional damage of dopaminergic neurons, long blocked by antipsychotics in the caudate nucleus. Especially when the drug is discontinued, these supersensitive striatal receptors respond excessively to the now unblocked dopamine. Acetylcholine is thought to have an opposing effect to dopamine in the extrapyramidal system.

Treatment of TD has been based on the postulated dopamine-acetylcholine imbalance and includes dopamine-depleting agents (reserpine, tetrabenazine, oxypertine, α-methyldopa, α-methyl-p-tyrosine) dopamine blockers (a variety of antipsychotic drugs including pimoside and clozapine), and cholinergic medication (choline, physostigmine). Antiparkinsonian drugs, L-dopa and psychomotor stimulants have been shown to worsen tardive dyskinesia symptoms. Other drugs used have been dilantin, antihistamines, deanol, vasodilators, amantadine (Symmetrel), lithium, antianxiety agents, sedatives, serotonin receptor blockers, serotonin synthesis inhibitors, tricyclic antidepressants, monoamine oxidase inhibitors, long-term dopa and low dose methyl phenidate.

It is quite remarkable how many drugs are said "to help" TD. A substantial number of patients have had their TD gradually disappear with the passage of many months. If a drug was administered in this period, this spontaneous improvement might have been falsely attributed to the drug. Undoubtedly this may explain why so many drugs are reported to benefit TD. Controlled studies in our laboratory have *failed* to show amatadine (Symmetrel) and deanol to be effective. In addition, we have found that a large placebo effect may accompany TD symptoms. To control for the spontaneous remissions, which occur in many patients, as well as for placebo effect, properly designed control studies must be done and uncontrolled findings interpreted with caution until therapeutic efficacy is proven.

Because TD treatment is often unsuccessful, the most effective means is prevention. The least possible antipsychotic dose needed should be given. All patients should be reexamined periodically to determine if they really need their drug. Every so often the patient should be examined for abnormal movements including those of the unprotruded tongue. It seems the syndrome is more likely to be reversible if discovered early.

In spite of the danger of TD, the patient who needs an antipsychotic should get it. Efforts should be made to limit the use of antipsychotics, particularly long-term antipsychotics, only to those patients who need them.

We would first recommend a trial of TD patients without medication for some extended period of time. Many patients will have their TD completely disappear. If not, the next drug we would suggest is reserpine. Occasionally, exacerbation of psychosis requires antipsychotic drug treatment. Reserpine has antipsychotic properties and we would recommend reserpine if it does the job. Of course, there are schizophrenics so severely affected that they must be maintained on more powerful antipsychotic medications. Rarely, patients have TD with such severity that they need an antipsychotic agent to suppress it. Despite the fact that this drug may be continuing to produce more of the undesirable changes, it does suppress the symptom. In rare instances, this is unavoidable. For preventing long-term TD in patients chronically on antipsychotic drugs, it is often helpful to taper the drug over several days and then discontinue it for a week. Such drug-free periods, which can be arranged every year or so, may provide a test to see if TD is present. If TD surfaces in such a period, then every effort can be made to manage the patient without using antipsychotic medication.

Convulsive Seizures

This rare side effect occurs mostly after treatment with chlorpromazine or promazine, and is related to high dose and rapid elevation. Seizures can occur after any antipsychotic. Epilepsy is not a contraindication to antipsychotic use, but warrants caution.

Autonomic Nervous System Toxic Effects

The probable mechanism involved is either α-receptor blockade or atropine-like action of the antipsychotics. Many effects disappear in 1 to 2 weeks and are more annoying and potentially disruptive to patient cooperation than dangerous.

Autonomic Nervous System Toxic Effects	
• Tachycardia	• Paralytic ileus
• Hypotension—dizziness or faintness	• Constipation, diarrhea, nausea, vomiting
• Dry mouth and oral moniliasis	• Bladder paralysis
• Blurred near vision	• Edema
• Nasal congestion	• Pupil—large or small
• Pallor	• Ejaculation inhibition

Hypotensive effects are predominantly postural and more commonly promazine- or chlorpromazine-induced, especially after parenteral use. Danger of falls exists in older people.

It is theoretically possible for epinephrine to produce primarily β-adrenergic effect and paradoxical hypotension in a patient who had a relative α-adrenergic blockade from phenothiazines. Therefore, norepinephrine may be safer in such patients.

Ejaculation inhibition most commonly follows thioridazine treatment and consists of a delay or complete blocking of ejaculation but does not interfere with erection. Unless patients are warned about this effect, they can become alarmed.

Allergic or Toxic Effects

Agranulocytosis

This rare side effect has a peak occurrence between three and eight weeks. Watch for it carefully because it can be fatal. The prevalence of true agranulocytosis is in the order of magnitude of 1:1,000,000 cases, but good data are not available.

This condition usually develops in a few days, and patients often have normal white blood cell (WBC) counts several days before its onset. The weekly blood count advised by some physicians for the first three months of phenothiazine therapy as a precaution is, therefore, ineffective, and not recommended.

Furthermore, the gradually declining WBC count (e.g., 5500 to 3500 in two weeks) is different from agranulocytosis and should not be confused with it. The best diagnostic tool is clinical alertness for the high fever and sore throat (with ulcerations) that are then found associated with a WBC count of below 500 and less than 2% polymorphonuclear leukocytes. You should not neglect blood counts, nor glibly assume that a patient's fever is merely a winter cold. A doctor who takes note of minor clinical symptoms and an attentive nurse are more important than is meaningless routine hematology.

This condition's pathophysiology is that of a toxic bone marrow reaction. The side effect seems more common after promazine or chlorpromazine than other phenothiazines, but the figures are poor.

Agranulocytosis occurs typically in older women. The antipsychotic should be discontinued. Treatment must be vigorous. Antibiotics are indicated after culture and sensitivities have been drawn. Other supportive measures may also be needed. If the initial phase is not fatal the WBC count will return to normal within 10 days.

Since agranulocytosis is, in some sense, an allergic reaction, individuals who have had an episode should not receive chlorpromazine again since a repeat episode would be expected.

Dermatoses

- *Systemic dermatoses*—Most often a maculopapular rash on face, neck, chest and extremities, a non-dose-related allergic reaction, occurs 2 to 8 weeks after treatment initiation. Occasionally, angioneurotic edema of eyelids, lips and hands ensues and rarely exfoliative dermatitis, which can endanger life and requires vigorous use of epinephrine, cortisone, aerosols and supportive measures.

  Approximately 5% of patients on chlorpromazine develop a skin rash, but, as with other side effects, such estimates' are inexact and often include all simultaneously occurring allergic dermatoses, drug allergies and non-medication dermatoses.

• *Contact dermatoses*—Can occur in nurses and others whose hands come in contact with phenothiazines.

• *Photosensitivity*—Direct sunlight is the energy source thought to act on chlorpromazine to produce free radicals, resulting in damage to the surrounding skin. Severe sunburn can occur after relatively mild exposure. Lesions most often occur in light-exposed areas and are sunburn-like and intensely erythematous. Most cases are caused by chlorpromazine. Other phenothiazines produce this side effect to a lesser extent or not at all.

Jaundice

The symptoms include a prodrome of fever, nausea, right upper quadrant abdominal pain and malaise, followed within a week by intense pruritus and then jaundice. Alcholic stools and dark urine are often present.

Jaundice usually occurs within the first month of treatment and is usually benign and self-limited in course.

The condition may or may not be visible; some patients have fever, abdominal pain and tenderness, but no yellow color. Others have abnormal liver function tests with no clinical symptoms. When unexplained fever occurs in patients on chlorpromazine therapy, consider obstructive jaundice, as well as agranulocytosis, as a possible cause.

Laboratory studies reveal elevated alkaline phosphatase, modestly increased serum glutamic oxaloacetic transaminase and elevated direct (conjugated) bilirubin with bilirubinuria. An allergic reaction is suggested by the lack of dose relationship, elevated blood eosinophils and subsequent positive challenger responses to chlorpromazine. The jaundice may be caused by small bile duct obstructions caused by a hypersensitivity reaction. Cross-sensitivity among phenothiazines is unusual.

The incidence of chlorpromazine jaundice is declining and most likely lies between 0.1 and 0.5%. Chlorpromazine seems to cause this liver disease more frequently than the other phenothiazines.

Metabolic or Endocrine Effects

Weight Gain

Patients do gain weight during phenothiazine treatment, perhaps most often from chlorpromazine. Little can be done except diet and exercise. Psychomotor stimulants can make schizophrenic patients worse. Molindone seems to be the only antipsychotic known not to cause weight gain.

Feminizing Effects

- *Galactorrhea and gynecomastia*—galactorrhea may follow antipsychotics, and is accompanied by amenorrhea. Galactorrhea probably results from increased prolactin secretion by the anterior pituitary. Other causes of nonpuerperal galactorrhea must be ruled out, such as Cushing's syndrome, hyperthyroidism, adrenal carcinoma, myxedema, testicular choriocarcinoma, Chiari-Frommel syndrome and nonacromegalic pituitary tumors.

  Gynecomastia in males is infrequent but can occur. Non-drug causes must be ruled out such as liver cirrhosis, malnutrition, Klinefelter's syndrome, exogenous hormone (e.g., estrogens), testicular tumors, pubertal changes and spinal cord lesions.

  Galactorrhea and gynecomastia are best handled by dose reduction, by changing to another drug, or both.
- *Amenorrhea*—menstrual irregularities occur and are common in women with psychiatric illnesses. Galactorrhea often accompanies this condition, suggesting decreased secretion of prolactin inhibitory factors as the mechanism.

  Amenorrhea should be an occasion for ruling out pregnancy; reduction of dosage is also warranted. Rarely, the particular drug should be discontinued. A false urine (not serum) A-Z test is sometimes associated.

Glucose Metabolism

Phenothiazines have a hyperglycemic effect in some patients, but cannot be considered as causing diabetes. However, they may precipitate an attack in predisposed patients. Nevertheless, phenothiazines can be used with caution in diabetic schizophrenics. Monoamine oxidase-inhibiting drugs *do* lower blood glucose. Use caution when combining these drugs with insulin or sulfonylurea derivatives. Neuropsychiatric patients, in general, have higher incidences of blood glucose abnormalities.

Body Temperature Alterations

Both hypo- and hyperthermia occur. Chlorpromazine was initially used to produce a therapeutic decline in temperature. The mechanism is both a central hypothalamic and a peripheral adrenergic blockade.

Hyperpyrexia has been said to be produced by antipsychotic agents. However, many psychiatrists feel that the rare episode of marked hyperpyrexia seen in psychiatric patients (temperature 108°F) may be the rare syndrome of lethal catatonia, unrelated to psychotropic drug medication. Since patients developed this syndrome long before the psychotropic drugs were discovered, the occurrence of this syndrome probably is unrelated to medication, and may be falsely attributed to it. In tropical countries where patients with infectious disease present markedly elevated temperatures, ice packs plus chlorpromazine is more effective in lowering a temperature than ice packs alone. It is well established that anticholinergics can predispose patients to heat stroke. In situations of high environmental heat, patients can develop common heat stroke, high fever, confusion progressing to coma and cessation of sweating. Rapid treatment by ice cold water, spray with fans or both, and vigorous massage is mandatory since these conditions are potentially fatal and constitute a medical emergency.

Miscellaneous Effects

Toxic Retinopathy

Thioridazine can produce pigmentary retinopathy in patients receiving 1200 mg or more daily. Fundal pigment appears clumped or rarified, and visual acuity diminishes. The patient notices a brownish discoloration of vision before the fundus shows dramatic changes. The onset is usually between treatment days 20 and 50. Thioridazine below 800 mg daily does not seem to be associated with this condition. Loss of visual acuity can proceed even to blindness. Most believe the retinal pigmentation abnormality to be irreversible, but visual acuity may be restored once thioridazine is stopped.

The arbitrary maximum dose of thioridazine is 800 mg per day. This allows a safety factor, since doses of 50 to 100% are required to produce the pigmentary retinopathy. If a patient needs more than this dose limit, a second antipsychotic can be added on top of the thioridazine, or a new antipsychotic can be substituted for thioridazine. If a patient is inadvertently placed on higher than normal doses of thioridazine, the patient should quickly be switched to another drug, and an eye examination should be performed.

Drug-Induced Skin/Eye Syndrome

Discoloration of sunlight-exposed skin areas, such as face, nose, back of hand and neck, begins with a tan or golden-brown color and progresses to slate gray, metallic blue or purple after long-term, high-dose chlorpromazine therapy. Because it often occurs in conjunction with corneal and lens opacities, whenever a "purple people" reaction is observed, the patient's eyes should be examined.

Skin discoloration following chlorpromazine treatment was noted in the mid-1950s, but not until 1964 did Greiner and Berry recognize a skin and eye syndrome after long-term, high-dose chlorpromazine treatment. The skin and eye deposits have not been shown to be identical side effects. Although they do occur with a fair frequency in the same patients, one can occur without the presence of the other. They both seem to be related to long-term, high-dose chlorpromazine therapy and to sunlight exposure.

Whitish-brown granular deposits in the eye occur roughly in the following sequence: anterior lens, posterior cornea, anterior cornea, conjunctiva, skin and, finally, possibly the retina.

Lens changes start with fine bilateral particles visible only by slit-lamp in the anterior capsular and subcapsular pupillary area. Eventually, a polar stellate granule becomes visible in the anterior lens. Investigators agree that lens and corneal deposits rarely, if ever, diminish vision and then only after they reach an extremely advanced stage.

This dose-related cumulative eye phenomenon most likely results from retention of a chlorpromazine-melanin complex. Usually, a minimum of 1000 g (not milligrams) of chlorpromazine is required, but a few cases of lower dosage have been reported (probably not lower than 550 g). The reaction is idiosyncratic, as well as dose-related, since all patients receiving sufficient amounts do not develop pigmentation.

Reported incidence of eye pigment deposits varies greatly, probably due to differences in dosage, climate, patient group and ophthalmologists' criteria for defining pathological conditions.

Ocular deposits due to advancing age, congenital conditions and other nonchlorpromazine factors must be eliminated. Incidences from less than 1% to over 30% have been reported in various hospital groups.

Diagnosis can be made by penlight, ophthalmoscope, or slit-lamp. Eye examination might be conducted before commencing extensive "mega" high-dose, long-term chlorpromazine therapy and then at regular intervals, varying with dose level.

Once visible, corneal and lens opacities are slowly and only partially reversible. Therefore, the best treatment is prevention through such measures as: minimizing maintenance chlorpromazine dosage, using drugs other than chlorpromazine, avoiding excessive sunlight. These measures result in significant skin pigmentation reversal, but only a moderate decrease in ocular pigmentation. Substituting another phenothiazine for chlorpromazine can maintain psychic improvement, while not adding to ocular and dermal pigmentation. Butyrophenones can also be substituted. Unfortunately, however, thiothixene (Navane) may produce similar corneal and lens effects.

It has been speculated that sunlight catalyzes chlorpromazine or chlorpromazine metabolites to form free radicals which may interact with melanin to form this pathology. The deposits are not normal melanin granules, but melanin-like, and the eye and skin pathophysiologies may not be similar.

Effects on the Newborn

Antipsychotics do not cause congenital malformations and so are not contraindicated in pregnancy. However, they can have extrapyramidal and other adverse effects on the newborn. A postnatal depression syndrome followed by agitation has been noted. The effects of chlorpromazine on the nursing infant are not significant.

Conclusions

The drugs presented below seem to have a higher incidence of the particular side effects listed. Remember, phenothiazines are, for the most part, safe drugs. Most side effects are mild and easily controlled. Serious side effects are rare.

Drug	Higher Incidence of Side Effect
Chlorpromazine	Agranulocytosis, jaundice, sedation
Fluphenazine, perphenazine, trifluoperazine, thiothixene, haloperidol, molindone, loxapine	Extrapyramidal effects
Thioridazine	Retinopathy, inhibition of ejaculation, sedation

WHAT YOU WANTED TO KNOW ABOUT SIDE EFFECTS BUT WERE AFRAID TO ASK: PATIENTS' ATTITUDES TOWARD DRUGS

Is the patient's attitude toward drugs important?

First you must realize that psychiatric patients discuss both good and bad drug effects with friends, family, ward staff and other doctors. Through these discussions, they influence each other. They are also influenced by magazines, and may even read medical journals and other technical literature to learn about the drugs they are taking. Caudill noted a "ground swell" phenomenon. Most hospitalized psychiatric patients do "well or poorly at a particular time." Side effects can be similarly contagious. They may also provide ways of getting the doctor to listen or serve as vehicles for covertly expressing anger. "Your drug has made be dizzy," or "It's given me a headache," may mean that your patient is angry. He thinks you are ignoring him or that you do not care.

What questions do you think a physician should ask himself when a patient complains about a side effect?

A mental checklist is helpful. For example, were the side effects present before beginning medication? A careful predrug evaluation is essential. But sometimes it fails to distinguish a symptom or a sign from a pre-existing physical disease. You can miss lenticular opacities and tardive dyskinesias in your predrug history. You may start a patient on drug X. Yet, he may already have side effect Y from drug Z, his previous medication.

Another important question which the physician should ask himself is whether the alleged side effect is a symptom of the psychiatric condition itself. Dry mouth, for example, can be caused by amitriptyline or depression. A patient may have a peculiar gait before you give him any medication at all. Careful observation, prior to prescription, can answer the question: Is the side effect due to an entirely separate cause?

Perhaps the patient has an allergy that is causing his skin eruptions. The antipsychotic drug may not be the sensitizing factor.

Some of the more common toxic reactions and their managements seem to be left out of many textbooks. Are they so easily treated or trivial that everyone knows how to handle them?

Absolutely not! In our experience as consultants, the number of questions asked us about these side effects precludes their triviality. They often cause patients to abandon or impulsively change their antipsychotic medications.

Drowsiness. In the case of psychotic students whose performance is threatened by drowsiness, we recommend a piperazine drug, halopcridol, thiothixene or loxapine. You can also assure your patient that the drowsiness will abate within 10 days. You can decrease the dosage or give as much of the dosage as possible at night. But do not prescribe amphetamines to counteract the drowsiness, especially for schizophrenics.

Dry Mouth. This common, distressing side effect can sometimes lead to monilial infection. Instruct your patient to chew sugarless gum or lozenges to avoid this infection. If severe dry mouth occurs, prescribe bethanecol chloride (urecholine) 25 mg. t.i.d. orally. Frequent mouth rinsing and reassurance that the side effect will subside is also beneficial. Bethanecol chloride has also been affective in relieving drug-induced bladder inhibition and constipation.

Does treating older patients present any special risks?

Yes, postural hypotension is particularly disturbing for this patient group. We recommend the piperazine phenothiazines instead of the aliphatics that more commonly cause this side effect.

How do you manage postural hypotension once it is present?

Postural hypotension is most severe during the first treatment week, especially the first thing in the morning. Warn your older patient to arise in gradual stages—sit up, dangle his legs, then stand. Explain the mechanism of orthostatic hypotension and that it is the most common cause of dizziness and weakness. When this side effect is severe, patients can faint and be badly injured. However, patients rapidly develop tolerance to it. You can also prescribe surgical elastic stockings to prevent blood pooling in the extremities.

What is the treatment of choice for drug-induced skin rashes?

Psychiatrists do not yet agree on a specific treatment. Most phenothiazine skin rashes are transient. If they are persistent or severe, switch to another drug. Cross-sensitivity is rare, so this management is usually feasible.

You could prescribe diphenhydramine or another antihistamine to alleviate itching, but we are not yet convinced that they are useful.

In addition, you must guard against the rare possibility of exfoliative dermatitis.

How is phototoxicity best managed?

The best way to handle this problem is by preventing it. Warn your patient against excessive sun exposure—especially in spring and summer. Painful sunburns can occur in a very brief time if your patients do not use sun-protective lotions, creams and broad-brimmed hats if they are exposed to the sun.

What do you do if your patient develops jaundice?

Terminate the drug, prescribe bed rest and, if necessary, start other antipsychotic agents immediately. If possible, wait until the jaundice subsides before prescribing a new antipsychotic drug.

Do phenothiazines and antiparkinsonian drugs cause blurred vision?

Yes, the mechanism is usually through mydriasis and cyclopegia. The blurring usually abates within one week, and is rarely serious. If your patient becomes agitated, reduce the dosage for a while. Also warn him about driving his car during this period.

Phenothiazines produce near vision blurring. If your patient's far vision is disturbed, look for another cause.

Sometimes 1% pilocarpine nitrate or 0.1% physostigmine eye

drops may help clear up the mydriasis, but probably not the cyclopegia. If difficulty in reading continues, using or changing glasses may help. We have found glasses particularly helpful.

Does glaucoma contraindicate phenothiazine treatment?

It does not in patients already being treated. Danger exists, however, for undiagnosed patients. The anticholinergic phenothiazines can precipitate an acute glaucoma attack. Before prescribing antipsychotic drugs, ask your patients about recurring blurred vision attacks, aches and pains in and around the eyes, or if they see colored rings around lights at night.

A positive family history usually exists for a patient with chronic (simple, open angle) glaucoma, but the acute angle closure type has no such built-in warning.

Which drugs cause urinary retention?

Phenothiazines, tricyclic antidepressants, antiparkinsonian (AP) drugs and monoamine oxidase inhibitors. Urinary retention can be serious, especially in older patients with prostatic hypertrophy. The additive anticholinergic properties of a phenothiazine-antidepressant-antiparkinsonian combination are particularly likely to cause this side effect.

We have not yet discussed in detail the parkinsonian extrapyramidal side effects caused by antipsychotic drugs. How do you manage these EPS?

A wide range of AP drugs are available for treating these EPS. You can also use antihistamines, such as diphenhydramine hydrochloride (Benadryl).

What, then, is the best treatment for akathisia?

To begin with, akathisia is the most common EPS. You can often mistake it for agitation, which is distressing to your patient. Unfortunately, it is occasionally refractory to AP medication.

If you have to use large amounts of AP drugs for treating akathisia, your patient can develop atropine-like toxic reactions. The optimal treatment may be moderate doses of AP agents and switching to another phenothiazine to alleviate this EPS. Diazepam is sometimes helpful.

You said dystonias are treatable with AP medication, didn't you?

Yes, intramuscular or intravenous AP drugs reverse acute dystonic states. So do diphenhydramine, diazepam, caffeine and amobarbital.

Do you believe in administering antipsychotic and AP drugs simultaneously? Or would you rather start drug treating with antipsychotics first, using AP medication only if you run into EPS?

The question of whether or not to use AP drugs remains unsettled to some degree (Table 3.10). There is a shift in the thinking of many physicians toward not using prophylactic AP drugs, unless there is some particular reason to do so. For example, some prefer not to routinely use them, but to restrict them to patients who have had extrapyramidal side effects in the past, or patients with a drug which has a high propensity to produce extrapyramidal side effects. In the past, some physicians have routinely used AP drugs. However, since opinion is divided, a recommendation cannot be made at this time. Some physicians still use prophylactic AP drugs in all patients, others never use it in any patients, and others, like ourselves, feel it should be used selectively. There is clear agreement on one point, however: patients should not be maintained on

Table 3.10
Antiparkinsonian (AP) Drugs*

Trade name	Generic name	Dose (mg)	Frequency/ day
Kemadrin	Procyclidine hydrochloride	5–10	1–4
Cogentin, Tremin	Benztropine methanesulfonate	1–2	1–3
Artane, Pipanol	Trihexyphenidyl hydrochloride	2–5	1–4
Akineton	Biperiden hydrochloride	2–4	1–4
Pagitane	Cycrimine hydrochloride	2.5–5	1–3
Disipal	Orphenadrine hydrochloride	50–100	1–4

* All of the above AP agents are synthetic anticholinergic drugs resembling atropine. No definitive studies exist comparing efficacy, so they can be used interchangeably. Most are short-acting and require oral or parenteral administration two or three times a day.

AP drugs for the rest of their lives. We feel that patients initially placed on antiparkinsonian drugs should have their drugs discontinued after 3 months of treatment. There have been a large number of studies of patients who have been routinely put on AP drugs; when these are discontinued, they do not develop extrapyramidal side effects, perhaps because they never would have suffered them anyway.

Remember that for many of the antipsychotic drugs, only 15 to 30% of the patients develop extrapyramidal side effects. In addition, patients become tolerant of the extrapyramidal side effects produced by the antipsychotics. Some who would experience extrapyramidal side effects in the first few weeks would not have them several months later. Since there is a large body of data showing that most people do not need AP drugs after 3 months, it follows that for most patients such drugs should be discontinued at about this time. Of course, patients developing extrapyramidal side effects during discontinuance should be treated with AP drugs. Studies on discontinuance of AP drugs sometimes are misinterpreted to mean that prophylactic AP agents do not work. These studies are not relevant to prophylactic medication since they are dealing with discontinuance of this drug in patients who have been on it for some period of time. To date, there is only limited literature on prophylactic medication, and one study showed that in patients treated with placebo and perphenazine, about 27% developed extrapyramidal side effects, whereas if AP drugs were added to perphenazine for prophylaxis, 10% developed extrapyramidal side effects. In other words, prophylactic AP drugs prevented more than 50% of the extrapyramidal side effects that would have occurred. Clear evidence against the use of routine AP drugs can be seen from the fact that only a minority of patients develop these side effects. Although the anticholinergic side effects are generally not a problem, they can, on occasion, rarely contribute to such side effects as bladder or bowel paralysis, dry mouth, blurred vision, mental confusion, and toxic psychosis (central anticholinergic syndrome). In addition, the medication is an added expense. There is no evidence that AP drugs prevent TD; nor is there any evidence that the AP drugs contribute to the development of TD. Since there is some evidence of a conflicting nature from the literature on animals, no conclusions can be reached at this time.

It has been suggested that the anticholinergic drugs interfere with the absorption of chlorpromazine and, hence, lower plasma levels. This could be one mechanism by which these drugs work to relieve parkinsonism, but, clearly, this could not account for the rapid response of such symptoms to intravenous anticholinergics. Thus, we can assume that such drugs directly antagonize the dopamine blockade in the central nervous system.

Once you have started a patient on AP drugs, when is the best time to withdraw treatment?

Many psychiatrists try to reduce or stop AP medication after several months, while continuing the antipsychotic drug. It is always a good practice to terminate unnecessary medication, because it is expensive and can be harmful. One more caution: once AP medication is stopped, be careful not to overlook insidious apathetic akinesia. You can easily miss it, as can the patient and his family, and it can be quite harmful to social and vocational adjustment. Finally, if you are going to withdraw both antipsychotic and AP medication, terminate the antipsychotic first. It has long-lasting effects, and phenothiazine-induced EPS and physiological upset can occur if APs are withdrawn first. Both medications should be tapered over a week or two.

References

Ayd, F. J., Jr.: The depot fluphenazines: a reappraisal after ten years' clinical experience. Am. J. Psychiatry *132*: 491–500, 1975.

Bishop, M. P., and Gallant, D. M.: Loxapine: A controlled evaluation in chronic schizophrenic patients. Curr. Ther. Res. 12:594–597, 1970.

Caffey, E. M., Diamond, L. S., Frank, T. V., et al.: Discontinuation or reduction of chemotherapy in chronic schizophrenics. J. Chronic Dis. 17:347, 1964.

Carlsson, A.: Antipsychotic drugs, neurotransmitters, and schizophrenia. Am. J. Psychiatry *135*:164–177, 1978.

Casey, J. F., Hollister, L. E., Klett, C. J., et al.: Combined drug therapy of chronic schizophrenics. Controlled evaluation of placebo, dextro-amphetamine, imipramine, isocarboxazid, and trifluoperazine added to maintenance doses of chlorpromazine. Am. J. Psychiatry 117:998, 1961.

Chien, C. P., Di Mascio, A., and Cole, J. O.: Antiparkinsonian agents and depot phenothiazine. Am. J. Psychiatry *131*:86–90, 1974.

Chouinard, G., Annable, L., Serrano, M., et al.: Amitriptyline-perphenazine interaction in ambulatory schizophrenic patients: A controlled study of drug interaction. Arch. Gen. Psychiatry 32:1295–1307, 1975.

Clark, M. L., Huber, W. K., Sakata, K., et al.: Molindone in chronic schizophrenia. Clinical Pharmacol. Ther. *11*: 680–688, 1970.

Clark, M. L., Huber, W. K., Sullivan, J., et al.: Evaluation of loxapine succinate in chronic schizophrenia. Dis. Nerv. Syst. 33:783–791, 1972.

Clark, M. L., Parades, A., Costiloe, J. P., et al.: Loxapine in newly admitted chronic schizophrenic patients. J. Clin. Pharmacol. 15:286–294, 1975.

Clark, M. L., Ramsey, H. R., Ragland, R.

E., et al.: Chlorpromazine in chronic schizophrenia. Behavioral dose-response relationship. Psychopharmacologia 18:260–270, 1970.

Clark, M. L., Ramsey, H. R., Rahhal, D. K., et al.: Chlorpromazine in chronic schizophrenia. Arch. Gen. Psychiatry 27:479, 1972.

Cole, J. O., Goldberg, S. C., and Klerman, G. L.: Phenothiazine treatment in acute schizophrenia. Arch. Gen. Psychiatry 10:246–261, 1964.

Cole, J. P., and Clyde, D.: Extrapyramidal side effects and clinical response to the phenothiazines. Rev. Can. Biol. 20:565, 1961.

Crane, G. E.: Tardive dyskinesia in patients treated with major neuroleptics: A review of the literature. Am. J. Psychiatry 124(Supp.): 40, 1968.

Curry, S. H., Janowsky, D. S., Davis, J. M., et al.: Factors affecting chlorpromazine plasma levels in psychiatric patients. Arch. Gen. Psychiatry 22: 209, 1970.

Curry, S. H., Marshall, J. H. L., Davis, J. M., et al.: Chlorpromazine plasma levels and effects. Arch. Gen. Psychiatry 22:289–296, 1970.

Davis, J. M.: Comparative dose and costs of antipsychotic medication. Arch. Gen. Psychiatry 33:858–861, 1976.

Davis, J. M.: Efficacy of tranquilizing and antidepressant drugs. Arch. Gen. Psychiatry 13:552, 1965.

Davis, J. M.: Dopamine theory of schizophrenia: A two-factor theory. In The Nature of Schizophrenia, (Wynne, L. C., ed.), Ch. 9, pp. 105–115, New York, John Wiley & Sons, Inc., 1978.

Davis, J. M., and Chang, S.: Does psychotherapy alter the course in schizophrenia? In Controversies in Psychiatry Ch. 13. (Brodies, K., and Brady J. P., eds.), New York, W. B. Saunders, 1978.

Davis, J. M., Ericksen, S. E., and Dekirmenjian, H.: Plasma levels of antipsychotic drugs and clinical response. In Psychopharmacology: A Generation of Progress (Lipton, M. A., DiMascio, A., and Killiam, K. F., eds.) New York, Raven Press, 1978.

Garver, D. L., Davis, J. M., Dekirmenjian, H., et al.: Pharmacokinetics of red blood cell phenothiazine and clinical effects. Arch. Gen. Psychiatry 33:862–866, 1976.

Garver, D. L., Dekirmenjian, H., Davis, J. M., et al.: Neuroleptic drug levels and therapeutic response: Preliminary observations with red blood cell bound butaperazine. Am. J. Psychiatry 134:304–307, 1977.

Goldberg, S. C., Schooler, N., Hogarty, G., and Roper, M.: Prediction of relapse in schizophrenic outpatients treated by drug and sociotherapy. Arch. Gen. Psychiatry 34:171–184, 1977.

Goldberg, S. E., Frosch, W. A., Drossman, A. K., et al.: Prediction of response to phenothiazines in schizophrenia: A cross-validation study. Arch. Gen. Psychiatry 26:367, 1972.

Gorham, D. R., and Pokorny, A. D.: Effects of phenothiazine and/or group psychotherapy with schizophrenics. Dis. Nerv. Syst. 25:77, 1964.

Greenblatt, M., Solomon, M. H., Evans, A. S., and Brooks, G. W., eds.: Drug and Social Therapy in Chronic Schizophrenia. Springfield, Ill., Charles C. Thomas, 1965.

Grinspoon, L., Ewalt, J. R., and Shader, R. I.: Schizophrenia: Pharmacotherapy and Psychotherapy. Baltimore, Williams & Wilkins, 1972.

Hanlon, T. E., Schoenrich, C., Frenck, W., et al.: Perphenazinebenzotropine mesylate treatment of newly admitted psychiatric patients. Psychopharmacologia 9:328–399, 1966.

Hirsch, S. R., Gaind, R., Rhode, P. D., et al.: Outpatient maintenance of chronic schizophrenic patients with long-acting fluphenazine double blind placebo trial. Br. Med. J. 1:633–637, 1973.

Hogarty, G. E., and Goldberg, S. E.: Drugs and sociotherapy in the aftercare of schizophrenic patients. Arch. Gen. Psychiatry 28:54, 1973.

Hogarty, G. E., Goldberg, S. C., Schooler, N. R., et al.: Drugs and sociotherapy in the aftercare of schizophrenic patients. Arch. Gen. Psychiatry 31:603–618, 1974.

Hogarty, G. E., Ulrich, R. F., Mussare, F., and Aristiqueto, N.: Drug discontinuation among long term, successfully maintained schizophrenic outpatients. Dis. Nerv. Syst. 37:494–500, 1976.

Hollister, L. E.: Complications from psychotherapeutic drugs. Clin. Pharmacol. Ther. 5:322, 1964.

Hollister, L. E., Overall, J. E., Meyer, F., et al.: Perphenazine combined with amitriptyline in newly admitted schizophrenics. Am. J. Psychiatry 120: 591, 1963.

Horn, A. S., and Snyder, S. H.: Chlorpromazine and dopamine. Conformational similarities that correlate with the antischizophrenic activity of phenothiazine drugs. Proc. Nat. Acad. Sci. U.S.A. 68:2325, 1971.

May, P. R.: Treatment of Schizophrenia. New York, Science House, 1968.

May, P. R. A., Tuma, A. H., Yale, C., et al.: Schizophrenia—a follow-up study of results of treatment II. Hospital stay over two to five years. Arch. Gen. Psychiatry 33:481–486, 1976.

National Institute of Mental Health Psychopharmacology Research Branch Collaborative Study Group: Short-term improvement in schizophrenia: The contribution of background factors. Am. J. Psychiatry 124:900–909, 1968.

Murphy, D. L., and Wyatt, R. J.: Reduced monoamine oxidase activity in blood platelets of schizophrenic patients. Nature 238:225, 1972.

Prien, R. F., and Cole, J. O.: High dose chlorpromazine therapy in chronic schizophrenia. Report of National Institute of Mental Health: Psychopharmacology Research Branch Collaborative Study Group. Arch. Gen. Psychiatry 18:482–495, 1968.

Prien, R. F., Levine, J., and Cole, J. O.: High dose trifluoperazine therapy in chronic schizophrenia. Am. J. Psychiatry 126:305–313, 1969.

Quitkin, R., Rifkin, A., and Klein, D. F.: Very high dose vs. standard dosage fluphenazine in schizophrenia. Arch. Gen. Psychiatry 32:1276–1281, 1975.

Smith, R. C., Tamminga, C., Haraszti, J., et al.: Effect of dopamine agonists in tardive dyskinesia. Am. J. Psychiatry 134:763–768, 1977.

Smith, R. C., Dekirmenjian, H., Davis, M. M., et al.: Plasma butaperazine levels in long-term chronic non-responding schizophrenics. Comm. Psychopharmacol. 1(1):319–324, 1977.

Smith, R. C., Tamminga, C., and Davis, J. M.: Effect of apomorphine on chronic schizophrenic symptoms. J. Neurol. Transmiss. 40(2):171–177, 1977.

Smith, R. C., Dekirmenjian, H., Crayton, J., et al.: Blood levels of neuroleptic drugs in non-responding chronic schizophrenic patients. Arch. Gen. Psychiatry (in press).

Spohn, H. E., Lacousiere, R., Thompson, K., et al.: Phenothiazine effects on psychological and psychophysiological dysfunction in chronic schizophrenia. Arch. Gen. Psychiatry 34: 633–644, 1978.

Steinbook, R. M., Goldstein, B. J., Brauzer, et al.: Loxapine: a double-blind comparison with chlorpromazine in acute schizophrenic patients. Curr. Ther. Res. 15:1–7, 1973.

Tamminga, C. A., Schaffer, M. H., Smith, R. C., et al.: Schizophrenic symptoms improve with apomorphine. Science 200:567–568, 1978.

Wijsenbeek, H., Steiner, M., and Goldberg, S. C.: Trifluoperazine: A comparison between regular and high doses. Psychopharmacologia 36:147–150, 1974.

Zeller, E. A., Boshes, B., Davis, J. M., et al.: Molecular aberration in platelet monoamine oxidase in schizophrenia. Lancet 1:1385, 1975.

chapter FOUR

Pharmacological Treatment for Mood (Affective) Disorders

DIAGNOSIS OF DEPRESSION

Depressive illness is more than a transient unhappy mood. There is a significant loss of interest in, and the ability to derive pleasure from, work, sex, friends, food, entertainment—in fact, from everything.

Major Depressive Disorder

Major Depressive Disorder, Single Episode

Major Depressive Disorder, Recurrent

Criteria
A. One or more Depressive Episodes
B. Has never had a Manic Episode

Manic Disorder

Manic Disorder, Single Episode

Manic Disorder, Recurrent

Criteria
A. One or more Manic Episodes
B. Has never had a Depressive Episode

Bipolar Affective Disorder

Bipolar Affective Disorder, Manic

Criteria
A. Has had one or more Depressive Episodes
B. Currently (or most recently) in a Manic Episode

Bipolar Affective Disorder, Depressed

Criteria
A. Has one or more Manic Episodes
B. Currently (or most recently) in a Depressive Episode

Bipolar Affective Disorder, Mixed

Criteria
A. Current (or most recent) episode involves the full symptomatic picture of both Manic and Depressive Episodes, intermixed or rapidly alternating every few days.
B. Depressive symptoms are prominent and last at least a full day.

Major Affective Disorders

Mania Episode

A. One or more distinct periods with a predominantly elevated, expansive or irritable mood which must be a prominent part of the illness and relatively persistent although it may alternate with depressive mood. Mood change is not due to substance intoxication.
B. The illness has had a duration of at least 1 week (or any duration if hospitalized) during which for most of the time at least three of the following symptoms have persisted (four symptoms if mood is only irritable) and have been present to a significant degree.
  (1) Increase in activity—either socially, work, or sexual, or physically restless.
  (2) More talkative than usual or pressure to keep talking.
  (3) Flight of ideas or subjective experience that thoughts are racing.
  (4) Inflated self-esteem (grandiosity, which may be delusional).
  (5) Decreased need for sleep.

(6) Distractibility, i.e., attention is too easily drawn to unimportant or irrelevant external stimuli.

(7) Excessive involvement in activities with lack of concern for potentially harmful consequences, e.g., buying sprees, sexual indiscretions, foolish business investments, reckless driving.

C. Not superimposed on either Schizophrenia, Schizophreniform Disorder, or a Paranoid Disorder.

D. None of the following dominate the clinical picture when affective symptoms are not present (i.e., symptoms in criteria A and B above).

(1) Preoccupation with a mood-incongruent delusion or hallucination (see definition below).

(2) Bizarre behavior.

E. Not due to any Organic Mental Disorder.

F. Not superimposed on Schizophrenia.

Note: A hypomanic episode is a pathological disturbance similar to, but not as severe as a manic episode.

Note: Subclassify as nonpsychotic or psychotic (delusions or hallucinations other than the simple hearing of a name called).

Depressive Episode

A. Loss of interest or pleasure in almost all usual activities and/or dysphoric mood, characterized by symptoms such as: depressed, sad, blue, hopeless, low, down in the dumps, irritable. This must be prominent and persistent, but not necessarily the most dominant symptom. It does not include momentary shifts from one dysphoric mood to another dysphoric mood, e.g., anxiety to depression to anger, such as are seen in states of acute psychotic turmoil.

B. Each of at least four symptoms have been present nearly every day for a period of at least 2 weeks.

(1) Poor appetite or significant weight loss (when not dieting) or increased appetite or significant weight gain.

(2) Insomnia or hypersomnia.

(3) Psychomotor agitation or retardation (but not mere subjective feelings of restlessness or being slowed down).

(4) Loss of interest or pleasure in usual activities, or decrease in sexual drive (do not include if limited to a period when delusional or hallucinating).

(5) Loss of energy, fatigability, or tiredness.

(6) Feeling of worthlessness, self-reproach or excessive or inappropriate guilt (may be delusional).

(7) Complaints or evidence of diminished ability to think or concentrate such as slowed thinking, or indecisiveness (not if associated with obvious formal thought disorder).

(8) Recurrent thoughts of death, suicidal ideation or wishes to be dead, or any suicide attempt.

C. Not superimposed on either Schizophrenia, Schizophreniform Disorder, or a Paranoid Disorder.

D. None of the following dominate the clinical picture when affective symptoms (A and B) are not present.

(1) Preoccupation with a mood-incongruent delusion or hallucination. Delusions or hallucinations whose content is not consistent with the themes of either personal inadequacy, guilt, disease, death, nihilism, or deserved punishment.

(2) Bizarre behavior.

Note: Subclassify as Not Psychotic or Psychotic, as above.

(3) With psychotic features: The clinician should specify whether the psychotic features are mood-congruent or mood-incongruent. (The non-ICD-9-CM fifth digit 7 may be used to indicate that the psychotic features are mood-incongruent; otherwise mood-congruence may be assumed.) In addition, the clinician may wish to specify whether the disorder is With Melancholia or Without Melancholia.

Mood-congruent psychotic features. Delusions or hallucinations whose content is entirely consistent with the themes of either personal inadequacy, guilt, disease, death, nihilism, or deserved persecution.

Dysthymic Disorder (Depressive Neuroses)

A. During the past 2 years has been bothered most of the time by symptoms characteristic of the depressive syndrome, but not of sufficient severity to meet the criteria for a Depressive Episode.

B. These are persistent or separated by periods of normal mood lasting a few days to a few weeks, but no more than a few months at a time.

C. During the depressive periods there is either prominent depressed mood (e.g., sad, blue, down in the dumps, low), or marked loss of interest or pleasure in all, or almost all, usual activities and pasttimes.

D. During the depressive periods there are at least four of the following symptoms:

(1) Insomnia or hypersomnia.

(2) Low energy level or chronic tiredness.

(3) Feelings of inadequacy, loss of self-esteem or self-depreciation.

(4) Decreased effectiveness or productivity at school, work, or home.

(5) Decreased attention, concentration, or ability to think clearly.

(6) Social withdrawal.

(7) Loss of interest in or enjoyment of pleasurable activities.

(8) Irritability or excessive anger (in children, expressed towards parents or caretakers).

(9) Inability to respond with apparent pleasure to praise or rewards.

(10) Less active or talkative than usual, or feels slowed down or restless.

(11) Pessimistic attitude towards the future, broods about past events or feels sorry for self.

(12) Tearfulness or crying.

(13) Recurrent thoughts of death or suicide.

E. Not due to any other mental disorder.

Chronic Hypomanic Disorder

A. During the last 2 years, has had some symptoms characteristic of the manic syndrome most or all of the time, but not of sufficient severity to meet the criteria for a Manic Episode (although Manic Episodes may also have been present).

B. The manifestations of the hypomanic syndrome may be relatively persistent or separated by periods of normal mood lasting a few days to a few weeks, but no more than 2 months.

C. During the hypomanic periods there is either elevated, expansive, or irritable mood.

D. During the hypomanic periods there are at least three of the following symptoms that are clear changes from usual or former self:

(1) Decreased need for sleep.

(2) More energy.

(3) Inflated self-esteem.

(4) Increased productivity, often associated with unusual and self-imposed working hours.

(5) Sharpened and unusually creative thinking.

(6) Uninhibited people-seeking (extreme gregariousness).

(7) Hypersexuality without recognition of painful consequences.

(8) Excessive involvement in pleasurable activities without recognizing the high potential for painful consequences, e.g., buying sprees, foolish business investments, reckless driving.

(9) Physically restless.

(10) More talkative than usual.

(11) Overly optimistic or exaggerates past achievements.

(12) Inappropriate laughing, joking, punning.

E. The symptoms in D result in some impairment in social or occupational functioning.

F. Absence of delusions, hallucinations, incoherence, derailment (loosening of associations).

G. Not due to any other mental disorder, such as Cyclothymic Disorder or partial remission of Bipolar Disorder.

Cyclothymic Disorder

A. During the past 2 years, has had numerous periods during which there were some symptoms characteristic of both the depressive and manic syndromes, but not of sufficient severity to meet the criteria for a Depressive or Manic Episode (although Depressive or Manic Episodes may also have been present).

B. The manifestations of the two syndromes may be separated by periods of normal mood lasting as long as months, or they may be intermixed, or they may alternate biphasically.

C. During the affective periods there is depressed mood or loss of interest or pleasure in all or almost all usual activities and pastimes, *and* an elevated, expansive, or irritable mood.

D. During the affective periods there are *both* symptoms of at least three of the following pairs of symptoms:

Depressive	Hypomanic
(1) Insomnia or sleeping too much	Decreased need for sleep

(2) Low energy or chronic tiredness	More energy than usual
(3) Feelings of inadequacy	Inflated self-esteem
(4) Decreased effectiveness or productivity at school, work, or home	Increased productivity, often associated with unusual and self-imposed working hours
(5) Decreased attention, concentration, or ability to think clearly	Sharpened and unusually creative thinking
(6) Social withdrawal	Uninhibited people-seeking (extreme gregariousness)
(7) Loss of interest in or enjoyment of sex	Hypersexuality without recognition of possibility of painful consequences
(8) Restriction of involvement in pleasurable activities, or guilt over past activities	Excessive involvement in pleasurable activities without recognizing the high potential for painful consequences, e.g., buying sprees, foolish business investments, reckless driving
(9) Feels slowed down	Physically restless
(10) Less talkative than usual	More talkative than usual
(11) Pessimistic attitude toward the future, or broods about past events	Overly optimistic or exaggerates past achievements
(12) Tearfulness or crying	Inappropriate laughing, joking, punning

E. Absence of delusions, hallucinations, incoherence, derailment (loosening of associations).

F. Not due to any other mental disorder, such as partial remission of Bipolar Disorder.

Aaron Beck, M.D., includes four components in depression: *affective* (sad; loss of gratification and emotional attachments); *motivational* (increased wishes for help; overestimating difficulties; expecting everything to turn out badly, resulting in reluctance to act; inability to anticipate pleasure, leading to a paralysis of will); *cognitive* (negative attidues toward the self, the world and the future; the interpretation of present experiences negatively); and *vegetative* (fatigue; loss of appetite and libido; and retardation).

The diagnosis of depression is made, in part, by eliminating schizophrenic illness, which shows such manifestations as (1) delusions of being controlled; (2) thought broadcasting, insertion or withdrawal; (3) hallucinations, unless they are clearly related to depressed or elated mood; (4) auditory hallucinations, in which a voice keeps a running commentary on the patient's behavior or thought, or in which two or more voices converse with each other; (5) marked formal thought disorder.

Course and Prognosis

Well-defined Onset

Acute or subacute onset is more frequent than gradual onset.

After a well-defined onset, the condition usually worsens to a maximum, followed by steady improvement until the episode is over. Attack duration is variable, but averages about 6 months for inpatients and three months for outpatients. The duration of an episode varies considerably.

Spontaneous Remission

Complete recovery from an episode occurs in 50 to 90% of cases eventually.

Recurrence

After a first attack, 40 to 80% of patients experience recurrences. After the first attack, most patients have a symptom-free interval lasting more than 3 years. After subsequent attacks, the symptom-free interval decreases, although each episode is about the same length.

Suicide

Approximately 10 to 15% of hospitalized manic depressives will eventually commit suicide.

Comparison with Schizophrenia

Depression, unlike schizophrenia, shows a high rate of complete recovery to any given episode.

Classification of the Mood (Affective) Disorders

While the term "depression" is vague and is used variously to refer to a symptom, mood, affect or illness, we still believe that discrete depressive syndromes with distinct prognostic and treatment consequences can be defined.

The following list includes commonly diagnosed syndromes (in addition to those already described which enable the clinician to term the patient clinically depressed) with features that distinguish one from the other.

Bipolar vs. Unipolar

It is important to distinguish between bipolar depressive disease and unipolar depressive disease. There are a variety of differences between the two disorders. For example, in bipolar patients, tricyclics or L-dopa can switch a patient from depression to mania. In addition, bipolar patients tend to come from families which have bipolar depressive illness and unipolar patients tend to come from families with unipolar depressive illness. Bipolar illness has an earlier age of onset.

Single vs. Recurrent

It is obviously important to distinguish between single versus recurrent episodes, particularly with respect to depressive disorder. If patients have first or second or even third depressions, they can go on later to have a manic attack and, hence become bipolar. A patient who has had many unipolar episodes is probably a true unipolar.

Psychotic vs. Non-Psychotic

In our view, psychotic should mean the presence of delusions and hallucinations. In the case of depression, delusions are generally of being unworthy, condemned, criticized, or physically altered. Severity should be a separate dimension and not confused with psychosis.

Severe vs. Mild

It follows that the severity should be evaluated separately, and classified separately from psychosis.

Involutional Psychotic Reaction

This diagnosis is usually used for patients over 45 years of age suffering from a first depression with agitation, somatic concerns, insomnia, guilt and anxiety. In the American Psychiatric Association's *Diagnostic and Statistical Manual of Mental Disorders* (DSM III), such patients are classified as Major Depression: Single Episode or Recurrent (respectively). This is no longer a separate diagnostic category in DSM III.

Schizoaffective Reaction

These patients have an acute picture resembling schizophrenia (sometimes with a mixture of manic and schizophrenic symptoms, and sometimes with a mixture of psychotic depression and schizophrenic symptoms) followed by recovery. (See section in Chapter 1 on schizoaffective schizophrenia.)

Concepts in Depression

Primary vs. Secondary

Primary—Depression occurs in a patient without previous non-affective illness.

Secondary—Depression occurs after a previous mental or severe physical illness (alcoholism, schizophrenia, anxiety neurosis, obsessive-compulsive neurosis, organic brain syndrome, etc.). Depression may come before, with, or after many diseases such as viral infections, infectious mononucleosis, pancreatic illness, and may be confused with hypothyroidism.

Endogenous Depression

Endogenous is an ambiguous term and has two meanings. One refers to depressions which come unexpectedly, and without explainable precipitants, as opposed to depressions which are reactive to an explainable precipitant. A second and more common usage as defined operationally by many psychiatrists, particularly the British, involves the following characteristics: (1) a depressive mood which is qualitatively different from the normal depressions of everyday life; (2) anorexia; (3) insidious onset; (4) duration of less than one year; (5) early morning wakening; (6) the absence of precipitants; and (7) absence of neurotic self-pity, irritability, hypochondriasis, and hysteria, etc.). There is a large overlap between which patients should be classified as endogenous vs. reactive and the classification of primary vs. secondary. Endogenous in the British scheme is essentially the presence of pure depressive symptoms and the absence of pre-existing neurosis. Endogenous depression implies a depression of a biochemical origin, while reactive depression implies a psychological origin. Since endogenous has so many meanings, it is not a particularly good term for the purpose of classification.

It is better to use the more unambiguous classification of depressive patients on the dimensions of (1) primary vs. secondary; (2) mild vs. severe; (3) the presence or absence of precipitants; and (4) psychotic and nonpsychotic. The term endogenous has some usefulness in a more general sense by implying a biological type of depression which does not have precipitants. A further difficulty with precipitants is that many depressions do have precipitants, but they seem less obvious in the severe and/or psychotic depression because the patient may be too sick to dwell upon them.

Retarded vs. Agitated

Retarded
- Thought and action unspontaneous and slow
- May be found in any depressive diagnostic subtype (not specifically the manic depressive)
- Presence or absence of retardation is important when predicting drug response (i.e., good response to tricyclic).

Agitated
- Excess of unproductive activity (e.g., handwringing, pacing) and vocal expressions of severe psychic pain. Much of this behavior (e.g., handwringing, cuticle picking) causes bodily pain, perhaps to distract from psychic suffering. Agitation is common in involutional depressives.

Certainly, many patients responding to antidepressants are thought to have a biologic component to their depression. However, psychological exploration reveals that many of these patients have psychological factors relating to their depression also. As such, we think psychological as well as drug treatment may be indicated. There are patients whose depression appears to be characterological and reactive in nature which does not appear to be in any sense biological. In some cases, drug treatment is ineffective but in some cases drug treatment does produce clinically significant improvements. In retrospect, it can be said that these patients may have, in some sense, a biologic depression. Psychiatry cannot separate apart drug responsive and drug unresponsive patients, biological and psychological patients. The DMS III nomenclature is entirely descriptive in intent. Although much uncertainty exists, a conceptual distinction can be made between the more biological, endogenous patient, and the characterological, reactive dysphoric type. We would emphasize that much needs to be done to clarify these issues.

Reactive (exogenous, situational, psychogenic or neurotic)
- Caused by external stress.
- Symptoms fluctuate according to psychological factors.
- Hysterical postures.
- Initial insomnia; worse in evening.
- Does not respond to electroconvulsive therapy (ECT).

One problem with this concept is that age has not been controlled for in the pertinent studies. Older patients have early-morning insomnia and anorexia (and are called endogenous). In some cases, reactive depressions become autonomous, do not respond to environmental relief (e.g., remarrying after divorce) and should then be treated as endogenous.

The Clinical Entity of Endogenous-Like Depression vs. Other Dysphorias

Endogenous-like depression—Patients experience a lack of present and anticipated pleasure. They feel a loss of competence that is continuous for days or even months. The capacity for enjoyment is absent or severely limited.

Dysphoria—Enjoyment is possible, given the right circumstances, but complaints about severe subjective distress and unhappiness are continuous. There are two types of dysphorias: chronic characterological and acute.

Dysphoric States

Reactive dysphoria is unhappiness following severe disappointment, lasting about two months in an otherwise normal personality. This is *not* a disease.

"Depressions" in neurotic and character disorders can take the form of

- Overly severe disappointment reactions in deviant personalities (tantrums, sulking, suicide threats).
- Passive-dependent reactions with dysphoric complaints. Such individuals suffer angry unhappiness and low self-esteem, but are able to enjoy themselves (you may have to deduce this since they often cannot admit it).
- Hysterical people are "brittle" and experience mood swings ranging from giddy elation to desperate unhappiness. They are rejection-sensitive and overly responsive to the environment. Their affects are shallow and characterized by rapid lability, rather than being fixed and sustained as in the depressed patient.
- Chronically disappointed and demoralized patients. They are unhappy, dissatisfied, preoccupied with losses, feel "short-changed," are emotionally labile, histrionic, demanding, complaining, clingingly dependent, irritable, angry, self-pitying, blame-avoiding, and hypochondriacal.

SHOULD ALL DEPRESSIVES BE MEDICATED?

The Debate

Controversy is greater here than about schizophrenia because indications for antidepressants in certain types of depression are not well defined. Also, depressives are usually more docile in their behavior than schizophrenics. They do not require chemotherapy to control intolerable behavior.

Con:

It has been said that drugs may interfere with psychotherapy, but empirical research has proved this to be false. A study of maintenance psychotherapy and/or drugs indicates that maintenance drugs prevent relapses of depression, but do not improve many aspects of psychological functioning. On the other hand, psychotherapy does have a substantial beneficial effect on the psychological functioning of the patient, but does not prevent relapse. Modern thinking on psychotherapy vs. drugs indicates that the two forms of treatments are complementary, and they may help the patient through different mechanisms. The tricyclic antidepressants treat or prevent the depressive illness, and psychotherapy assists with psychological problems. Of course it is possible that in some sense the therapies may potentiate each other, or at least be additive. Indeed, one recent study of mild outpatient depressions shows that the antidepressant effect on both are greater than either alone so their effects are additive.

Pro:

Depression can be a serious clinical entity which may lead to suicide, and is recurrent. The patient should be given as painless an experience as possible to prevent a subsequent episode from provoking self-destructive behavior.

On the average, approximately 40% of depressions remit spontaneously in about one month. With tricyclic drug treatment, about 70% remit during this same time period. Adding a second drug treatment in patients not responding to the first increases the improvement rate from 70 to 85%. Thus, the patient's chance for rapid recovery is approximately doubled if somatic treatments are used.

Speed of treatment is important. If the patient is only ill for a brief time, perhaps a month, she/he can be temporarily excused from work and family obligations. However, an illness of a year or more can result in job loss and permanent family disruption.

THE WORK-UP

The First Steps

Depression can result from drugs like reserpine, propranolol, methyldopa, amphetamines, other stimulants (so-called post-amphetamine depression), oral contraceptives, and sometimes from marijuana, alcohol or hallucinogens.

Previous episodes of depression or mania and possible precipitating factors should be questioned. A family history of depression and response to treatment should, where possible, be discovered.

Depressives tend to be older than schizophrenics. Thus, in addition to a careful medical and somatic therapy history and physical and laboratory tests, pay close attention to the following problems.

Cardiovascular Problems

Watch out for congestive heart failure, severe postural hypotension, myocardial infarction, precipitation of cardiac arrhythmias, particularly pre-existing conduction disturbances such as heart blocks when giving antidepressant medications. These agents must be given cautiously and in low dosage to the elderly or to those with serious cardiac pathology. Baseline electrocardiograms (ECGs) can be helpful occasionally.

Prostate-Urinary Difficulty

Urinary retention is more likely to occur in patients with an enlarged prostate.

Constipation

Take a history of the patient's bowel habits, and estimate any effect that the depressive illness may have before attempting to accurately determine aggravation by the antidepressant drug.

Acute Glaucoma

You can precipitate acute glaucoma with drug treatment in patients with unsuspected narrow-angle glaucoma. Ask them about recurring attacks of blurred vision, pain around the eyes and colored rings around lights. Antidepressant medications are not contraindicated in chronic simple glaucoma.

Predrug or routine weekly laboratory tests are probably unnecessary. In the elderly, pay attention to cardiovascular status, or other medical problems.

Other Dangers to Anticipate

Use tricyclic antidepressants (TCAs) with caution in patients who have a history of schizophrenia or presenting symptoms. Hallucinations and delusions may be precipitated in such individuals.

Drug Interactions

Tricyclic antidepressants (including Doxepin) and antipsychotic drugs antagonize the antihypertensive effect of guanethidine (Ismelin) or clonidine.

To produce its antihypertensive effect, guanethidine must be taken up by the norepinephrine-containing neurons which innervate the vascular system. This uptake mechanism is the same mechanism as involved in the uptake of norepinephrine, and is blocked by both the tricyclic antidepressants and many antipsychotic agents.

If a patient is already receiving a monamine oxidase inhibitor (MAOI), stop the drug and observe the patient for a minimum of 1 week before beginning TCA treatment. Failure to do so can rarely result in high fever, convulsions and even death, although recently some have suggested that the dangers of this combination have been exaggerated.

Suicide

TCA overdose is much more life-threatening than phenothiazines. You must be able to differentially diagnose TCA poisoning. The clinical picture reflects atropine toxicity, tachycardia, dilated pupils, flushed face, etc. TCA overdose alters the ECG, producing arrhythmia and widening of the QRS complex. Confirm the diagnosis by analyzing the gastric lavage material. Treat with gastric lavage and paraldehyde or diazepam for convulsions. Physostigmine can be useful to counteract the anticholinergic toxicity of TCAs, including tachycardia and delirium. However, cardiac problems are the critical medical problem.

WHICH DRUG FOR WHICH PATIENT?

Most seriously depressed patients and many with mild depression should be treated with an antidepressant. The antidepressant class of choice, for almost all patients in initial treatment, is the tricyclic antidepressants which in general, are more effective than the MAOIs. The criteria for treating mild depression with medication is not well developed. The general absence of research to define indications for treatment means the clinician must depend on his clinical experience. Primary depressions and endogenous depression classically respond to tricyclics. Since there is a high correlation between these two classifications, this is to be expected. Those patients who respond well tend to have functioned normally prior to onset, and to have had a sudden acute onset of depressive affect, early morning awakening, feelings of pessimism, difficulty making decisions, retardation, an inability to feel pleasure from things which were usually enjoyable, and the absence of pre-existing mental disease such as alcoholism, schizophrenia or neurosis. There is some evidence to suggest that retardation predicts good response to imipramine. Good responses are seen in both psychotic and neurotic depressions; however, some psychotic depressions seem resistant to tricyclics. There is evidence that some delusional patients may not do particularly well with imipramine so that the addition of an antipsychotic and/or ECT may be indicated. Agitated patients respond to antipsychotic drugs such as thioridazine, thiothixene, perphenazine or chlorpromazine, so the addition of these drugs for short periods of time can be helpful as an adjunct to the tricyclics.

There is no clear guideline for determining the preferred treatment. Agitated depressed patients respond well to tricyclics so that it is not always necessary to add an antipsychotic. We would tend to use tricyclics if the depression is the predominant problem (Table 4.1).

There is clear indication for tricyclics in mild primary depressions if there is any evidence that these are persistent depressions. Amitriptyline and doxepin are the most sedating tricyclics, followed by imipramine, whereas the least sedating is protriptyline. Desimpramine and nortriptyline fall between imipramine and protriptyline. The desirability of sedative side-effects is a factor to consider in choosing a tricyclic. If a patient is having trouble sleeping, a sedating tricyclic can be used with most, or all, of the daily dose given at night.

If a patient fails to respond to tricyclics, and about 30% do not respond, it is important to determine whether the patient is taking his medication. The most important cause of failure to respond is non-compliance by the patient. The next consideration is dose adjustment and the plasma level. This will be discussed in a section on plasma levels, but the therapist should make an attempt at arriving at the optimal dose. If you are satisfied that the patient is receiving an optimal dose and he still fails to respond, the next question involves determining what drug to switch to.

As mentioned above, some depressions may be norepinephrine depressions, while others may be serotonin depressions. Although this theory has not yet been proven, it follows that if a patient fails on the drug thought to affect serotonin depressions, namely amitriptyline, it would be reasonable to try the patient on a drug known to affect norepinephrine depressions, such as imipramine, desipramine, nortriptyline, or protriptyline. Similarly, if a patient fails to respond to the four drugs thought to be more potent

Table 4.1
Classification of Drugs Used in the Treatment of Depression

Drug	Average dose (mg)
Tricyclic derivatives (TCA):	
Imipramine (Antipress, Imavate, Imipramine, Janimine, Presamine, SK-Pramine, Tofranil)	150–300
Desipramine (Pertofrane; Norpramin)	150–250
Amitriptyline (Amitril, Amitriptyline, Elavil, Endep)	150–300
Nortriptyline (Aventyl, Pamelor)	50–150
Protriptyline (Vivactyl)	10–60
Doxepin (Adapin, Sinequan)	150–300
Trimipramine (Surmontil)	75–200

Monamine oxidase inhibitors (MAO):	*Stimulants:*
Hydrazines	Amphetamine
Isocarboxazid (Marplan)	(Benzedrine)
Phenelzine (Nardil)	Dextroamphetamine
Nonhydrazines	(Dexedrine)
Tranylcypromine (Parnate)	Deanol (Deaner)
Withdrawn from U.S. market	Methamphetamine
Iproniazid (Marsilid)	(Amphedroxyn;
Pheniprazine (Catron)	Dexosyn)
Etryptamine (Monase)	Methylphenidate
Nialamide (Niamid)	(Ritalin)
New antidepressants not available in U.S.:	
Noxiptylin(e) (Agedal)	60–300
Melitracen(e) (Dixeran)	75–250
Monochlorimipramine (Anafranil)	3.75–200
Dimethacrin(e) (Istonil)	150–225
Dibenzepin (Noveril)	160–640
Iprindole (Tertran)	
Nomifensine	
Mianserin (Bolvidon)	
Amexapine	
Maprotiline	
Vilozazine	

antidepressants for norepinephrine depression, then amitriptyline would be indicated. Doxepin is not a well-studied drug in this regard, so predictions cannot be made at this time. This will increase the percentage of responders to 80%. If one tricyclic fails, the second tricyclic not infrequently does the job. About 50% of tricyclic failures will respond to ECT; some tricyclic non-responders also respond to MAOI treatment.

Other attempts to relieve depression include combining tricyclic antidepressants with lithium, T_3, Tryptophan, monoamine oxidase inhibitors, or sleep (or REM) deprivation. It has been reported and verified by the same group that the addition of T_3 for 5 days to tricyclics may shorten the time response of the tricyclic and, in some cases, it will be effective treatment for resistant depressed patients. Although this has been replicated by the same investigators, elsewhere there has been one failure to replicate this finding. More work is clearly needed. Methylphenidate does increase tricyclic plasma levels, but the same purpose can be accomplished by administering a higher dose.

"Depression" in Neurotics and Character Disorders

Hysteroid Dysphoria

TCA can produce negative results (racing thoughts, somatic distress, depersonalization, mania). Sometimes, such results cannot be accurately predicted, as in patients with an hysterical personality suffering from a clinical depressive illness. These persons display symptoms suggestive of both hysteroid dysphoria and neurotic depression. A TCA trial is indicated, but be prepared for negative psychogenic and even alarming results due to the patient's histrionic nature. Since you cannot predict which patients will respond positively, a therapeutic trial with TCAs is indicated for many. MAOI therapy is sometimes effective with such patients. They diminish the reactive dysphoria and the fruitless, unrewarding, self-destructive romantic involvements.

Reactive "Depressions" (Disappointment Dysphorias)

These painful conditions are self-limited and usually remit within two months. They can be associated with extreme subjective distress, and should be managed by supportive psychotherapy and small doses of an antianxiety agent.

The great majority of depressed patients have precipitating events in both primary and secondary depressions. This is not a good criteria in itself for the prescription of medication. Some patients who have mild depressions from some environmental events should be handled psychologically and not receive drugs. The exact criteria to separate those who should receive drugs from those who should not receive drugs has not been developed by research at this time. Certainly some mildly depressed patients should receive drugs and clinical judgment is indicated here. Many British psychiatrists feel that MAOIs are specific for hysterics with secondary depression. Carefully controlled studies document their usefulness in outpatient depression.

Demoralization

Demoralized people feel incapable or incompetent and, thus, avoid test situations. However, they are able to experience pleasure, especially in a setting with few demands. You can best manage them initially by accurate diagnosis, followed by supportive psychotherapy (suggestion, persuasion and identification with the therapist). Drug treatment does not play a major role.

Bereavement

When grieving, the sufferer is preoccupied with the lost object. Thus, bereavement can be distinguished from agitated depression in which the patient is preoccupied with his *own* psychic pain. One obvious factor in the differential diagnosis is the duration of suffering.

Do not use antipsychotic agents, antidepressants or barbiturates in managing the bereaved. If severe insomnia is present, we prefer to use an antianxiety agent. If a more severe state results (e.g., agitated or retarded depression, mania, psychosis, acute panic state), treat it accordingly. It is our experience that patients who have a serious depression precipitated by a loss cannot effectively grieve until they have recovered from their depression.

Geriatric Depression

Geriatric patients who are retarded, confused, uncooperative, irritable, sloppy or socially deteriorated may be so, in large measure, because of depression. Unfortunately, this diagnosis is often overlooked. Give adequate TCA cautiously. You are making a grave error if you give up on such a patient as organically damaged when he can, in fact, be helped.

This syndrome can be called "pseudosenile depression." These patients are not overtly depressed but, rather, have symptoms of senility, such as urine incontinence, confusion, etc. With TCA treatment, the senile symptoms may disappear. The patient can sometimes resume a productive role in society, rather than deteriorating on the chronic ward of a state hospital and progressing to an early death. For these patients, TCAs can be life-saving.

TCA: PRESCRIBING PRINCIPLES AND EFFECTIVENESS

TCA Effectiveness

In most controlled studies, these drugs are found to be superior to placebos with an overall improvement rate of 70%, versus 40% for placebo (Table 4.2). However, about 30% of patients do not show even moderate improvement on TCA treatment.

Most of these studies were done prior to the determination of the dose range necessary for recovery of some patients. For example, imipramine (Tofranil) and amitriptyline (Elavil) were initially recommended in a dose range of 75 to 150 mg. More recent experience indicates that the proper dose ranges from 75 to 300 mg. Had more adequate doses been used in these studies, the drug placebo difference would have been greater.

No TCA is clearly statistically superior to the parent compound, imipramine, in efficacy or speed of onset. Some studies show amitriptyline to be superior, yet this may be a dose-response artifact. Most studies show that all the tricyclic antidepressants are, on the average, equally effective. Demethylated derivatives are equal in speed of action to imipramine and amitryptyline.

Endogenous depressions probably respond to drugs better than do reactive ones. This often-made statement is a little misleading. Better response means "as opposed to placebo" in each case. The statement should therefore read: "Tricyclic antidepressant outperforms placebo in endogenous depression by a substantial margin, but they are only somewhat more likely to improve reactive depressions than placebo."

Even though TCAs are less effective for treating reactive depressions, the prognosis is much better than for endogenous depressions.

TCAs are not effective for treating normal sadness or lifelong depression. Normal sleep patterns can be restored by TCAs in depressed patients. Barbiturates make depressed patients sleepy, but do not cause the restorative phase of deep sleep to increase to normal levels.

Table 4.2
Clinical Evaluation of Antidepressant Treatment

Treatment	Drug more effective than placebo	Percent of studies in which		
		Treatment more effective than imipramine	Treatment equal to imipramine	Imipramine more effective than treatment
Imipramine (Tofranil, others)	68% (38)		—	—
Amitriptyline (Elavil, others)	82% (11)	29%	71%	0
Nortriptyline (Aventyl, Pamelar)	100% (4)	0	0* (7)	0
Desipramine (Norpramin; pertofrane)	60% (5)	0	86% (7)	14%
Protriptyline (Vivactil)	100% (2)	0	100% (2)	0
Tranylcypromine (Parnate)	67% (3)	0	100% (3)	0
Phenelzine (Nardil)	57% (7)	0	57% (7)	43%
Isocarboxazid (Marplan)	33% (6)	0	60% (5)	40%
Chlorpromazine (Thorazine)	100% (3)	0	100% (3)	0
Thioridazine (Mellaril)	—	0	100% (1)	0
Chlorprothixine (Taractan; Solatran)	—	0	100% (1)	—
Maprotiline (Ludiomil)	50% (4)	0	100% (10)	0
Amphetamine	0 (3)	—	—	—
ECT	88% (8)	43%	57% (7)	0

* Nortriptylene = amitriptyline in three studies.
Also 12 studies showing maprotiline exactly equal to amitriptyline.

Stages in TCA Treatment

Dosage

For our purposes, the milligram dosage of imipramine or amitriptyline is used below as an example, but conversion to another TCA is easy.

The rapidity of dosage increase depends upon the patient's age, medical status, severity of depression and whether or not he is hospitalized.

In medically healthy, young, severely depressed patients, 50 mg three times a day from the day of onset, gradually increased to 300 mg daily, constitutes an adequate trial. At times, you can exceed these numbers, especially for outpatients, but be cautious. A critical dosage exists for each individual patient, and this number must be reached for clinical response to occur. A general guideline is 3.5 mg of drug per kilogram of body weight, but the blood level achieved varies 8-fold from one patient to another. At least four studies show a relationship between blood level and clinical outcome with imipramine.

The existing controlled studies on the relationships between antidepressant plasma level and therapeutic response have been summarized in the following charts and graphs. The findings agree that if plasma levels of imipramine are low (less than 180 ng/ml), more subjects fail to respond. If plasma levels are high (greater than 240 ng/ml), the patient is apt to have an adequate plasma level for clinical response (Fig. 4.1). In the intermediate plasma level clinical response is uncertain. There is an inverted U-shaped relationship between plasma nortriptyline levels and clinical effectiveness (Fig. 4.2). One study finds that if plasma levels are very low (less than 50 ng/ml), there is failure to respond. The other studies were directed only to high dosage. Here, many studies agree that there is an upper end to dose effectiveness, but disagree about exactly where it is. Note that the time plasma levels were collected differs slightly among the studies. Such conventions must be worked out in order for the results to be clinically applied. Figure 4.2 gives the reader a better feel for the relationship between plasma level and therapeutic efficacy. This is more accurate than Figure 4.1 which gives an arbitrarily chosen number to reflect the upper and lower end of the therapeutic window. For protriptyline, there is considerable disagreement about the location of the ther-

		0 - 180	180 - 240	+240
Glassman	R	6	19*	
	NR	16	1	
Reisley	R	1	1	10
	NR	17	4	4
Martin	R	0	2	2
	NR	3	1	3
Muscettola	R	2	0	3
	NR	4	4	1

$$0 - 180 \quad 180 - 240 \quad +240$$

Plasma Levels (ng/ml)

Figure 4.1. Plasma levels vs. clinical response of patients treated with imipramine. R, responder; NR, non-responder. * Author gave plasma levels only as 180 and above.

apeutic window in the two studies performed (Fig. 4.3). Similarly, with amitriptyline there is some agreement that there is a dosage below which patients do not respond, but disagreement as to where the upper limit of the therapeutic window is located (Fig. 4.4). More work is needed to define the therapeutic window in order that plasma levels be clinically useful. Not only must the therapeutic window's existence be established, but it is necessary for laboratories to agree on its exact location. It is hoped that our graphs will help the reader place a given plasma level within perspective. Again, we would emphasize that plasma levels differ widely among individuals due to differences in the rate of metabolism in the liver. The clinician must adjust the dose for each patient individually to achieve maximum benefit with minimal side effects. Accurately determined plasma levels can occasionally

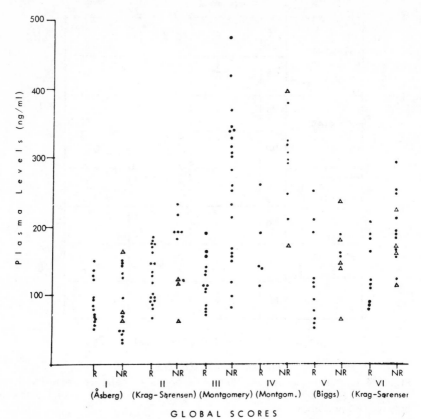

Figure 4.2. Nortriptyline plasma levels *vs.* global scores. R, responder; NR, non-responder; △, partial response.

aid in dose adjustment when the literature provides enough data to make sense of the number obtained and the likelihood of therapeutic response to that particular drug. We believe the best way to get a feel for plasma levels is not through arbitrarily selected numbers defining the upper or lower end to the therapeutic window, but by placing a given plasma level in the context of the data which we have presented graphically. (See references on Plasma Tricyclics.)

Although TCAs are usually given three times daily, the long duration of their action warrants a single dose one hour before sleep. Only oral ingestion seems justified, although some claim faster intramuscular results. Imipramine has a half-life of 14 hours, desipramine 20 hours, and amitriptyline 35 to 66 hours.

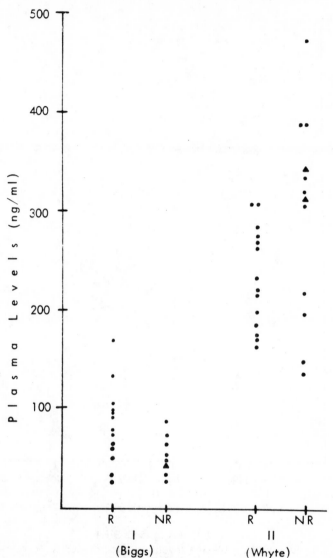

Figure 4.3. Protriptyline plasma levels *vs.* global scores. R, responder; NR, non-responder; △, partial response.

Combined Antidepressant-Antianxiety for the First Week

Roche has recently introduced a fixed combination of chlordi-azepoxide and amitriptyline for the treatment of mixed anxiety

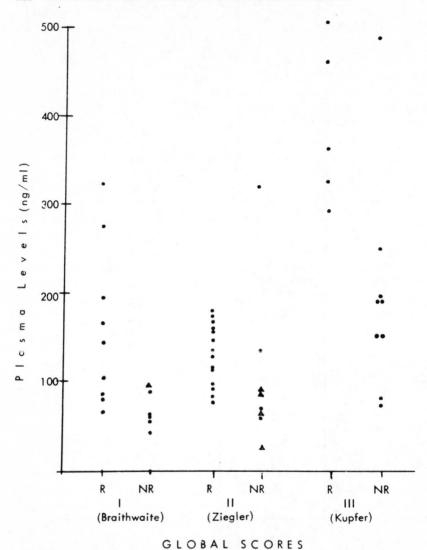

GLOBAL SCORES

Figure 4.4. Amitriptyline plasma levels *vs.* global scores. R, responder; NR, non-responder; △, partial response.

and depression in outpatients. They support the efficacy of this combination by results from a double-blind, multi-center collaborative study comparing their combination (trade name Limbitrol, which consists of 10 mg of chlordiazepoxide plus 25 mg of amitriptyline) to amitriptyline by itself, chlordiazepoxide by itself and placebo. In this study, 279 outpatients were evaluated. Chlordiazepoxide and amitriptyline are sedative drugs that have some antianxiety properties which improve insomnia and psychic and somatic anxiety. Given that chlordiazepoxide and amitriptyline each have sedative properties, it would be expected that they have additive effects in calming patients. Indeed, the combination does produce more improvement on items from the Hamilton Depression Rating Scale such as insomnia, agitation, and somatic and psychic anxiety during the first week of treatment.

Whether the increased improvement in one week results from the combined antianxiety properties of two sedative drugs, or reflects an added antidepressant effect, is unclear. However, the combination did produce greater improvement in the Depression Inventory on items such as pessimism, dissatisfaction, and guilt at 1 week. By the end of four weeks, most of the advantage of the combination was gone and amitriptyline alone was just as effective on many of the measures, and slightly, but not significantly, surpassed the combination on certain items.

Hare (1971) did two small studies of 20 outpatients with mixed anxiety-depression, comparing the combination against amitriptyline alone. In the first study, the combination was superior on several measures after 1 week. By week 3, the degree of improvement from both was more similar, and the initial difference had largely disappeared. In the second study, the results of the combination were quite similar to amitriptyline by itself. However, the statistically significant improvement on some measures still persisted for the combination. Haider (1967) studied seriously depressed inpatients and measured results only at three weeks, finding the combination to be superior to amitriptyline alone. Rickels et al. (1970) studied 243 mild to moderately depressed outpatients and found the combination, as well as each individual drug, superior to placebo. Because he only evaluated his results at 2 and 4 weeks, they cannot be compared to those of the Roche collaborative study after one week. Also, he did not compare amitriptyline-chlordiazepoxide to each drug separately so it is not possible to decide if the combination is superior to one or the other alone (i.e., he did not isolate the theoretically meaningful comparison statistically, namely, the contrast of amitriptyline as the combination).

It is clear that the addition of chlordiazepoxide (Librium) to a tricyclic does not interfere with its therapeutic action. There is some evidence available from the two studies cited here that it may be helpful during the first week of treatment. However, one study did not find it to be superior even at that time, and another failed to study its effectiveness during the first week. Additional evidence is needed to reach a firm conclusion. By three weeks, the combination no longer appears clearly superior.

Tricyclic Maintenance

There have been seven double-blind studies testing the efficacy of maintenance tricyclics in preventing relapse. The patients in the first two studies were initially treated with ECT and then placed on either placebo (or an active placebo) or treated with mainte- nance tricyclics, which prevented relapse (Seager, Kay). In the five other studies, patients were initially treated with tricyclics and then treated with placebo or a maintenance tricyclic with the intent of preventing relapse. These studies also showed that main- tenance tricyclics prevented relapse (see Table 4.3—note combined statistical test). In patients who have recurrent depressive disease there is clear evidence that a prophylactic medication should be prescribed. Of course many depressed patients have one episode and never have a relapse. These patients would not be candidates for long-term maintenance medication. How to determine exactly who should get continued drug treatment has not been defined, but the clinician must consider the number of depressive episodes and their severity in making the decision regarding the benefits of prophylactic medication as opposed to the risks. Lithium also prevents unipolar relapses, as well as relapses of bipolar patients. (See the section for lithium for discussion of the use of lithium in recurrent unipolar depression.)

Differences Among TCA:

Differences among TCAs including biochemical properties:
Imipramine (Antipress, Imavate, Imipramine, Janimine, Presa- mine, SK-Pramine, Tofranil).
Desipramine (Pertofrane; Norpramin)—the demethylated ver- sion of imipramine. (See Selected References on Maintenance Antidepressants.) A study comparing DMI and amitriptyline found less initial dry mouth, dizziness, blurred vision, constipation and sedation in DMI-treated patients. This may be useful in patients

Table 4.3
Placebo vs. Tricyclics for Prevention of Relapse of Recurrent Depression

Investigators	Number of patients who relapse or remain well on placebo or drug	
	Placebo	Drug
Prien *et al.*		
Relapse	24	17
Well	2	10
Mindham *et al.*		
Relapse	21	11
Well	21	39
Klerman *et al.*		
Relapse	27	6
Well	40	33
Coppen *et al.*		
Relapse	5	0
Well	11	13
Quitkin *et al.*		
Relapse	6	5
Well	2	3
Seager and Bird		
Relapse	11	2
Well	5	10
Kay *et al.*		
Relapse	24	8
Well	27	26

$p = 2 \times 10^{-9}$ (Fleiss, 1973).

who do not tolerate anticholinergic side effects.

Amitriptyline (Amitril, Amitriptyline, Elavil, Endep)—More sedating and hypnotic than imipramine and possibly more effective.

Nortriptyline (Aventyl, Pamelor)—The demethylated amitriptyline.

Protriptyline (Vivactyl)—Produces the least sedation of any TCA.

Doxepin (Sinequan; Adapin)—Claims of special tranquilizing properties have been dropped due to FDA insistence; has been used successfully mostly for mild depression or for mixed anxiety depressive states in outpatients (see Table 5.4).

New Antidepressants

Several new antidepressants have been extensively investigated. Trimipramine was found to be as effective as imipramine in several studies and has just been released in the United States. Opipromol consists structurally of an imipramine-type nucleus with a perphenazine side chain. It has been shown to be more effective than a placebo, and approximately equal to imipramine.

The recently developed antidepressant Maprotiline has been extensively researched in double-blind studies. There is no doubt from four double-blind controlled studies, considered as a group (two of which found maprotiline clearly superior to placebo and two of which found trends in this direction), that maprotiline is an effective antidepressant ($p = .001$ combined). Its efficacy, which is comparable to standard tricyclics, such as imipramine or amitriptyline, has been extensively documented. Ten investigations showed that maprotiline was exactly equal to imipramine in therapeutic effectiveness, and 12 studies showed that maprotiline was exactly equal to amitriptyline in therapeutic efficacy. We have reviewed this data from the point of view of statistical power. Since a large number of subjects were studied in double-blind studies, power considerations indicate that this data provides convincing evidence that Maprotiline is exactly equal in therapeutic efficacy to the standard tricyclics. Specifically in these carefully designed trials, 2078 patients were randomly assigned to either maprotiline or a standard tricyclic, usually imipramine or amitriptyline. In combining data in four-fold tables, where those patients who had moderate improvement, or better, were contrasted with those who did less well, the results indicated that 660 patients receiving maprotiline did well and 247 had minimal improvement, no change or worse outcome. The corresponding figures for standard tricyclic were 640 and 255, respectively. In percentage terms, 73% of the patients did well with maprotiline and 72% with standard drug. Similarly, incoming data by the method of Fleiss indicates that there is no difference whatsoever in efficacy between maprotiline and standard antidepressants.

Amexapine is another thoroughly investigated drug which has been shown to be safe and quite effective in a large number of double-blind studies.

Nomifensine has been extensively studied in Europe and South America and also has been investigated in a substantial number of double-blind studies where it has been compared to standard antidepressants and/or placebo. This body of data demonstrate that nomifensine is an effective antidepressant, comparable in efficacy to the standard antidepressants. It is a safe, non-sedating drug with a relatively low incidence of anticholinergic side effects. These three drugs have been extensively investigated and under active consideration by the FDA for release at the time of this writing. Mianserin has been shown to be an effective antidepressant. It is not an uptake or MAO inhibitor, but does increase norepinephrine turnover. There are other experimental antidepressants, such as the norepinephrine uptake inhibitor vilozazine, as well as 5-hydroxytryptamine uptake inhibitor, under clinical investigation.

ECT vs. TCA

ECT is more effective than TCA, which in turn is more effective than other antidepressants according to most studies (See Tables 4.4 through 4.6).

Table 4.4
The Efficacy of ECT vs. Simulated ECT (or Placebo)

Investigator	Number of patients who show a good or poor response		
	Response	ECT	Simulated ECT
Brill	Good	12	2
	Poor	6	6
Ulett	Good	28	14
	Poor	15	26
Fahy	Good	12	8
	Poor	5	9
Wilson	Good	6	3
	Poor	0	3
Harris	Good	2	1
	Poor	2	3
Shepherd (MRC)	Good	2	1
	Poor	2	3
		ECT	Placebo
Shepherd (MRC)	Good	49	23
	Poor	14	37
Greenblatt	Good	65	43
	Poor	5	24
Kiloh	Good	24	3
	Poor	3	25

$p = 1 \times 19^{-18}$.

Table 4.5
Efficacy of ECT vs. Tricyclics

Investigator	Number of patients who show a good or poor response to ECT or tricyclics		
	Response	ECT	Tricyclics
Harris	Good	12	3
	Poor	3	12
Wilson	Good	9	13
	Poor	1	3
Bruce	Good	21	16
	Poor	1	10
Shepherd (MRC)	Good	49	42
	Poor	12	19
Fahy	Good	12	10
	Poor	5	6
Greenblatt	Good	65	71
	Poor	5	28

$p = 4 \times 10^{-7}$.

Indications for ECT

Because of its rapid action and effectiveness, many clinicians begin severely suicidal patients directly on ECT. Those exhausted from malnutrition may be started directly on ECT. After four weeks, if adequate-dose TCA fails, you can try ECT.

Disadvantages of ECT

Relapse is common, but this is also true with all antidepressant drug therapies. Confusion, amnesia and recent memory loss are all results of ECT. Attempts to diminish these side effects have been made by using unilateral rather than bilateral ECT. Unilateral ECT is equally effective to bilateral, but produces only very minimal memory impairment.

ECT causes temporary mental confusion and memory loss. Some psychiatrists have wondered whether ECT might effect a permanent, but subtle, form of brain damage. Studies have generally found no brain damage after ECT, but we cannot rule out the possibility of a subtle impairment in some patients. General anesthesia is required. Since ECT alone does not prevent relapse, patients with recurrent disease need a prophylactic drug anyway.

Drug Advantages

There is no confusion, amnesia, memory loss nor any need for general anesthesia. Patients can often continue working.

Table 4.6
Effectiveness of ECT vs. MAO Inhibitors

Investigator	Number of patients who show a good vs. poor response to MAO inhibitors or ECT		
	Response	ECT	MAO inhibitors
Harris	Good	2	0
	Poor	2	4
Shepherd (MRC)	Good	49	19
	Poor	14	41
Greenblatt	Good	65	30
	Poor	5	42
Kiloh	Good	24	14
	Poor	3	12

$p = 7 \times 10^{-19}$.

When is ECT Ineffective?

- Mild, long-term depressions with hypochondriasis
- Chronic characterological depression
- Patients in whom anxiety is a primary problem

SIDE EFFECTS OF TCAs

Central Nervous System Effects

- Fine tremor (epinephrine-like, as opposed to coarse phenothiazine parkinsonism)
- Angry states
- Mania: TCAs can sometimes convert a depressive episode into a manic episode; with bipolar patients, TCAs can sometimes convert a depressed episode into a manic episode. This side effect should be watched for particularly in patients who have had previous episodes of manic illness, hypomania, who have had a family history of bipolar illness, or who have had a previous drug induced manic episode.
- Precipitation of hallucinations and delusions in latent schizophrenics
- Atropine-like psychosis

Tricyclic antidepressants can also cause an organic psychosis characterized by florid visual hallucinations, confusion, plus loss of immediate memory and orientation. The atropine-like properties of the TCAs are produced by the central anticholinergic syndrome (so-called atropine psychosis). It disappears generally within a day with discontinuance of the tricyclic. Evidence that it is a central anticholinergic syndrome is provided by its reversal by physostigmine (an agent which increases brain acetylcholine).

Autonomic Nervous System—Primarily Anticholinergic

- Glaucoma.
- Sweating.
- Postural hypotension, tachycardia and cardiac arrhythmias
- Urinary retention and paralytic ileus (rare); *caution*: patients with prostatic hypertrophy

Cardiovascular Changes

Tricyclic antidepressants (more often in overdose, rarely at therapeutic levels) can cause arrhythmias, blood pressure changes, direct depression of the myocardial muscle, anticholinergic activity (atropine-like tachycardia) or effects on adrenergic neuron (uptake inhibition of norepinephrine and epinephrine). The tricyclic antidepressants produce a quinidine-like effect on the heart. It follows that toxic effects of tricyclics and quinidine are additive, so there could be a problem in placing patients who are already on quinidine-like drugs on tricyclic antidepressants, or vice versa. Particular caution is indicated in using tricyclics in patients with preexisting heart block, since in overdose situations and occasionally at therapeutic levels, the tricyclic drugs slow conduction time.

ECG changes usually are of the reversible T wave variety. TCAs can exacerbate pre-existing conduction blocks, while producing an anti-arrhythmic effect on ectopic beats.

Sudden deaths have been reported in the Aberdeen study, but are not confirmed by the Boston Collaborative study. Treat elderly cardiac patients with TCAs for their depression, but cautiously, using lower than customary amounts, more gradual dosage increment, and careful monitoring of postural hypotension.

Sedative and Hypnotic Properties

Clinically depressed patients respond poorly to barbiturates and other hypnotics and are seldom relieved of insomnia, especially early morning awakening, by hypnotics alone.

Amitriptyline possesses sufficient hypnotic properties that if a fair amount of the patient's daily medication is given before bedtime, a good night's sleep is assured. Doxapine and amitriptyline are the most strongly sedative of the tricyclics, followed by imipramine, desipramine, nortriptyline, and finally protriptyline, which is the least sedative.

MONOAMINE OXIDASE INHIBITORS

Efficacy

MAOIs are either equal to or less effective than TCAs in most controlled trials with typical endogenous depression, but they are never superior to TCAs. However, in cases where tricyclics have failed and severe depression, dysphoria or neurasthenia exist, they are worth a try. The British find MAOIs effective in younger, non-hospitalized "atypical" depressives with marked anxiety, who may have hypochondriasis, irritability, agoraphobia, social phobia or who complain of lack of energy. They emphasize the need for adequate length of a clinical trial (six or more weeks) and proper dosage. Phenelzine was found to exceed placebo only at 60 mg daily and not at 30 mg. English investigators attribute MAOI failures in America to inadequate length of the clinical trial, too-low dosage, and selection of severe, hospitalized, endogenous depressives, rather than anxious, anergic, depressive, outpatient responders. Robinson, an American, has supported their contention. (See Table 4.7 for summary of studies. See also references on Monoamine Oxidase Inhibitors.)

Side Effects

Liver damage is extremely rare with hydrazine MAOIs, but severe parenchymal destruction can occur. Other problems are postural hypotension, a long duration of side effects, hypertensive crises, throbbing headaches, and flushing.

Agents Producing Hypertensive Crises

- Cheddar (or any high-tyramine) cheese (cottage cheese and cream cheese are safe).
- Certain beers and chianti wine.
- Chopped chicken livers (tyramine).
- Yeast products (e.g., Bovril used in gravies; Marmite).
- Sour cream and yogurt.
- Broad beans (fava beans)—due to L-dopa in the pods.
- Pickled herring (tyramine).
- Chocolate.

Table 4.7
Inpatient Studies Comparing Phenelzine and Placebo

Investigators	Patients	Dosage/duration	Summary of results

Robinson et al.	33/44 ph* completed
	27/43 pl completed
	depression with anxiety, phobia, and somatic concerns
		45–75 mg ph (58.5 mg mean), 6 weeks
		pl, 6 weeks
			Psychiatrist Rating _ph_ _pl_
			Definitely Im- 21 10
			  proved
			Possibly Improved 8 10
			No Change 3 5
			Worse 8 11
			                 $p = .02$

Ravaris et al.	49 of 62 completed
	14 ph, 60 mg
	16 ph, 30 mg
	19 placebo
	Matched age, sex, length of illness
	Depressed mood, anxiety, phobia, somatic concerns, coping problems
	23–81 years
		30 mg, 60 mg ph
		Placebo
		6 weeks
			Psychiatric Rat- _ph(60mg)pl_
			  ing
			Definitely Im- 10 4
			  proved
			Possibly Im- 1 6
			  proved
			No Change 3 9
			Worse 2 2
			            $p = .03$
			60 mg > pl for total depression, anxiety, hypochondriais, agitation, psychomotor change
			No difference ph (30 mg) and pl

Johnson and Marsh	39 slow acetylators completed 33 fast acetylators completed Neurotic depression	45–90 mg/day ph Placebo 3 weeks, 1st part of study	Improvement on weekly severity ratings Slow acetylators ph > pl $p = .0018$ Fast acetylators ph = pl $p = .077$
Lacelles	40 atypical anxious-depressives with atypical facial pain (20 ph) (20 pl)	4 weeks (before crossover) 45 mg/day Placebo	Improvement facial pain _ph_ _pl_ Market Improvement 6 1 Improvement 0 6 No Change 5 9 Worse 0 4 Significant differences on both facial pain and depression ratings

Table 4.7 (cont.)

Investigators	Patients	Dosage/duration	Summary of results		
Rees and Davis	20 patients (13 endogenous, 4 reactive, 3 mixed)	ph—90 mg, 3 weeks pl—3 weeks	Complete Improvement Marked Improvement Moderate Improvement Slight/No change Worse Moderately Worse	Ph 5 5 4 5 0 1	Pl 1 2 4 9 3 1	p = .006
Shepard (MRC)	61—ph 61—pl 40-69 yrs old	60 mg 4 weeks	Improved No Improvement	Ph 19 23	Pl 31 28	p = .60
Raskin et al.	44/110 ph completed 38/111 pl completed 36% psychotic 17% schizoid 51% neurotic 37-40 yrs old	45 mg—5 weeks Measures taken when off drugs two weeks	Ph = Pl			p = .50†
Greenblatt et al.	Severe depressed, mixed diagnosis (20% schizo) State hospital	60 mg (+15 optional) 8 weeks	Improved No Improvement	Ph 23 25	Pl 40 27	p = .14
Hare et al.	43-day hospital depressions	30 mg 2 weeks	Ph > pl on anxiety = on depression			p = .05†
Agnew et al.	Mixed, included schizo 4 Nardi 5 Pl	45 mg, 3 weeks	Much Improved Slight Improvement No Change Worse	Ph 2 1 0 1	Pl 0 0 4 1	p = .12
Klerman	Severe depressed Part of non-treatment study	3 weeks	Improved No Improvement	Ph 5 1	Pl 0 5	p = .013

* ph, phenelzine; pl, placebo.
† Probability approximated.

- Drugs: amphetamine, dextroamphetamine, methylamphetamine, ephedrine, dopamine, L-dopa, phenylpropanolamine (in proprietary cold preparations), any drug containing sympathomimetic compounds.

Treat the hypertensive crisis with a short-acting α-adrenergic blocking agent, such as phentolamine (Regitine), IV 5.0 mg, or 50 mg chlorpromazine IM. Do not use meperidine [phetidine (Demerol)]. Patients can be given several 100-mg chlorpromazine tablets to carry which can be taken in the event of a severe, throbbing headache.

Hypotension can occur. The mechanism is that false neurochemical transmitters (e.g., octopamine) are built up in sympathetic nerves during MAO inhibition.

Hyperpyrexic reactions are rare (e.g., high temperatures up to 108°F). Susceptible patients are those taking MAO inhibitors and then a high intramuscular dose of TCAs, or patients taking TCAs and MAOs in larger than normal amounts in a suicide attempt. The reactions are characterized by a high fever and excitement that progresses to coma and death. This side effect does not seem to occur when TCAs and MAOs are combined in low doses as the therapeutic treatment is given in gradual increments. This drug combination is used in England with some success, but is seldom used in the United States due to the extreme hazards of the interaction—hyperpyrexia and death. The combination may be useful for research by physicians skilled in psychopharmacology when dealing with a resistant depressed patient. However, for routine use by psychiatrists or family physicians, we do not recommend it. Hyperpyrexia, coma, excitation and fatal toxic reactions can also occur when MAOI patients are given meperidine (Demerol). The hyperpyrexia reaction can also occur in patients on MAOIs who are given amphetamines or tranylcypromine (parnate). Parnate has amphetamine-like properties, is metabolized to amphetamine, inhibits MAO, and inhibits the reuptake of biogenic amines. Hyperpyrexic reactions have been reported in patients who have been receiving tricyclics and parnate. Just which properties of parnate are particularly important in producing this reaction is unclear, but special caution should be called for when using parnate and tricyclic antidepressants, either sequentially or concomitantly, such as by leaving a longer period of time between stopping one drug and starting another.

STIMULANTS

Stimulants have no value in treating severe depression and are detrimental in schizophrenics, but it has been well established by many double-blind studies that you can prescribe them for hyperactive children. They are also effective in treating narcolepsy. The brief use in carefully selected cases of fatigue is possibly justified in the opinion of some clinicians. Psychiatric patients, especially psychotics, should not ingest these drugs for dieting. Although these stimulants are safe for hyperactive children, they can be associated with serious side effects and psychological dependency in adults.

Side Effects and Dangers

- Tenseness.
- Irritability.
- Dry mouth.
- Palpitations.
- Insomnia.
- Assaultiveness.
- Panic states.
- Hallucinations.
- Paranoid delusions.
- Post-drug depression.
- Habituation.
- Abuse.

LITHIUM CARBONATE (ESKALITH; LITHANE; LITHONATE) FOR TREATING MANIC DEPRESSIVE PSYCHOSIS

Manic vs. Schizoaffective State

Manic

Predominantly elated, expansive or irritable mood.
- Overactive
- Racing thoughts and pressure of speech that resists interruption
- The lack of need for sleep
- Elated, boastful, elevated mood
- Distractability

Inflated self-esteem (grandiosity which leads to a decreased need for sleep), excessive involvement in activities without recognizing painful consequences (e.g., buying sprees, sexual indiscretions, foolish business ventures, and reckless driving).

Schizoaffective

- Conceptual disorganization
- Unusual or bizarre thoughts
- Purposeless, stereotyped, symbolic or odd acts
- Hallucinations

At times, schizoaffective patients cannot be distinguished from "atypical manics," because typical manics respond well to lithium and schizoaffectives sometimes do not. This differential diagnosis is important.

How to Administer Lithium

The Work-Up

Take a careful medical history. Relative contraindications for lithium include kidney and cardiovascular disease, severe debilitation, low-salt diet, diuretics, excess sweating, diarrhea, old age and brain damage.

Laboratory tests needed are baseline T3, T4, and TSH (also palpate the thyroid); CBC (leukocytosis often accompanies lithium use); creatinine clearance and urinalysis; 24-hour urine volume; ECG and electrolytes in appropriate patients; (water deprivation urine concentration test sometimes useful).

Absorption, Distribution and Excretion

Lithium is rapidly absorbed, reaching maximum blood levels in from one to three hours. The peak is sometimes associated with nausea, vomiting, vertigo, muscular weakness and a dazed feeling. If this happens, give with meals. These discomforts subside in 30 minutes. Lithium is distributed throughout the total body water.

▶   **Lithium is absorbed rapidly and excreted by**   ◀ **the kidney.**

Blood determinations should be done 12 hours *after* the last dose (e.g., in the morning, before the first dose). Failing to do so can give distorted readings.

Because lithium is excreted via the kidneys, they must be functioning normally. One-half the lithium dosage is eliminated in 24 hours, but this process is slower in the elderly. More drug is retained when salt intake is low. Consequently, patients on low-salt diets, diuretics or those excessively perspiring tend to have toxic reactions on normal doses. Normal dietary NaCl is sufficient, and salt tablets are unnecessary.

Dosage. Administer lithium orally three times a day. Acute manics may require higher doses than patients on prophylaxis. It is often advisable to treat manic patients or atypical manics with lithium alone. If a response is achieved by lithium alone, this is an indication that lithium is the drug of choice for maintenance. Response to antipsychotics is non-specific. If a patient is treated with both lithium and antipsychotics, it is not known whether maintenance should be with one or the other.

Therapeutic dosage phase refers to the acute manic and should only be administered when the patient is hospitalized. Generally, six to twelve 330-mg tablets are given daily. Give lower doses to the elderly and adjust initially to plasma level.

Measure blood levels every two to three days to achieve the therapeutic dose level of approximately (0.8 to 1.2 milliequivalents (mEq) per liter. Do not exceed 1.6 mEq per liter or toxicity may occur.

In 1 week to 10 days, the acute manic episode subsides, and the lithium dosage must be cut somewhat. Failure to do so makes the patient toxic, since he may no longer tolerate the therapeutic amount. However, this has not been proven.

A 4 to 10 day lag period occurs before the therapeutic dose takes effect. During this period, you may have to combine a phenothiazine or butyrophenone with the lithium (then discontinue antipsychotic).

Maintenance Phase. An average dose of 600 to 1500 mg is required to achieve a blood level of 0.8 to 1.0 per liter. During this period, first determine blood levels once a week until stable, and then once every month.

Efficacy

No consensus exists about the mechanism of lithium's action. We do know, from controlled studies, that lithium is effective in about 70% of acute manics in ten days to two weeks. Due to the lag period, severe manics are difficult to manage with lithium alone. Indeed, in treating the acute manic, antipsychotic drugs are equal in efficacy to lithium. Many clinicians combine lithium and antipsychotic agents for the initial treatment phase. Some believe that lithium is superior, and that phenothiazines merely suppress manics, while lithium converts them to normal, but such thinking requires further verification.

Prophylaxis

Many consider lithium's main benefit to lie in prevention, rather than in treatment during the acute phase. Excellent evidence exists showing manic attacks to be decreased in frequency with maintenance lithium use (see Tables 4.8 and 4.9).

Patients with recurring depressive or manic depressive disease should be treated with maintenance lithium. Do not prescribe long-term lithium treatment lightly; it has a preventive action, indeed. Table 4.9 indicates the results of eight controlled studies. In studies that select for lithium-sensitive patients, lithium almost completely prevents relapse, while in studies where patients are not so carefully selected, lithium prevents substantially more relapses than does placebo. On the average, lithium reduces relapse by about one-quarter to one half. These results firmly establish this; the probability that this would occur by chance is about 2×10^{-34}. Lithium is effective in preventing both unipolar and bipolar disease (see Table 4.9).

Since Table 4.9 lumps bipolar and unipolar depressions, we constructed a table which insofar as possible separate these two subtypes out. As can be seen from this table, the evidence for lithium in bipolar disease is quite unequivocal. There is more controversy in regard to lithium prophylaxis of depressed episodes in unipolar depression, since a smaller number of patients have been studied. The most carefully controlled studies are those of Dunner, Baastrup, and Coppen, and their co-workers, but there is also information contributed by the International Collaborative Study and the study of Persson. Although these latter two studies are not as rigorously controlled as the others, because of the smaller number of patients, we will combine data from all of the studies. When considered in total, combining data with the statistical test of Fleiss, there is unequivocal evidence that lithium does prevent recurrence in unipolar depression. We can also ask the question as to whether the degree of prophylaxis of lithium in

Table 4.8
Effectiveness of Lithium vs. Placebo in Preventing Relapse

Investigators*	Patients in lithium group		Patients in placebo group		Significance†
	No. relapsed	No. not relapsed	No. relapsed	No. not relapsed	
Baastrup et al.	0	45	21	18	$p = 2.0 \times 10^{-9}$
Coppen et al.	3	24	33	3	$p = 4.0 \times 10^{-11}$
Hullen et al.	1	17	6	12	$p = 4.4 \times 10^{-2}$
Mendlewicz et al.	12	24	27	9	$p = 4.0 \times 10^{-4}$
Prien et al.	53	48	94	10	$p = 1.0 \times 10^{-9}$
Prien et al.	26	19	36	3	$p = 2.6 \times 10^{-4}$
Melia; Cundall et al.	7	9	13	3	$p = 3.3 \times 10^{-2}$
Persson et al.	11	22	25	8	$p = 5.7 \times 10^{-4}$
Dunner	22	16	34	9	$p = 3.4 \times 10^{-2}$
Quitkin	2	6	6	2	$p = 7.8 \times 10^{-5}$

* Most of the studies used a noncrossover design with random assignment and blind evaluation; however, the study of Cundall and associates used a crossover design, and Persson's study used a matched design (control patients were matched with lithium patients).

† By Fisher exact test. Overall significance $p = 2 \times 10^{-34}$.

bipolar depression is the same as the degree of prophylaxis in unipolar depression, i.e., irrespective of the number of patients studied: Is lithium as effective in preventing relapse in unipolar patients as in bipolar patients, or vice versa? In essence, some method of arriving at a correlation coefficient between the number of relapses on lithium and non-lithium, and having taken lithium or placebo is required. This data is expressed in Table 4.9 and indicates that the degree of prophylaxis is about the same in both types of affective disturbance. This data should be accepted in the context of the relatively small numbers of patients studied and also the fact that two of the studies reviewed are not as well controlled as the other three. It is important to remember also that this data is derived from patients who had many relapses and as such applies only to this population. How well it generalizes to patients who had a relatively smaller number of relapses is undeterminable at this time. In interpreting any data from research studies, you must always ask yourself how this data, arrived at from one population, generalizes to the patient in question. We feel it is effective in this condition; there is no data to define

Table 4.9
Lithium Prevention of relapse

Investigators	Bipolar patients (I and II)*		Unipolar depressions†	
	Placebo	Lithium	Placebo	Lithium
Baastrup et al. (1970)				
Relapse	12	0	9	0
Well	10	28	8	17
Prien et al. (1973)				
Relapse	93	47	14	13
Well	24	72	2	14
Persson (1972)				
Relapse	11	5	14	6
Well	1	7	7	15
Coppen et al. (1978)				
Relapse	21	3	12	1
Well	0	14	3	10
Fieve et al. (1976, 1978)				
Relapse	25	14	9	8
Well	4	10	5	6
Quitkin et al. (1978)				
Relapse	2	0	4	2
Well	1	3	1	3

* $p = 1 \times 10^{-21}$.
† $p = 1 \times 10^{-8}$.

whether lithium is necessarily any more effective in unipolar depression than are the tricyclics. The degree of prophylaxis achieved is slightly higher, but it may be that the populations studied had a better prognosis for drug treatment. More work needs to be done to define the role of lithium in prophylactic unipolar disease.

Lithium *is not* approved in the *Physician's Desk Reference* for use in prophylaxis of *unipolar* depression. Lithium *is* approved in the Physician's Desk Reference prophylactically for use in *bipolar* illness. There would be no problem in using lithium in patients previously diagnosed as unipolar, if criteria could be found to change the diagnosis to bipolar, such as the finding of a family history of bipolar illness, or the presence of previous mood swings. These patients may not meet the criteria of bipolar I, but could be considered bipolar II, or there may have been a previous drug-induced manic episode or hypomanic episode.

Depression

Although there is "suggestive evidence" for the efficacy of lithium in acute bipolar depression, there is general pessimism about the effectiveness of lithium in unipolar depression, so we would be particularly skeptical about this indication. More work needs to be done on lithium in the treatment of bipolar depression. There is not enough work to make a definitive statement about its use in treating the acute depressive episode in a bipolar patient. Since some evidence exists of lithium's effectiveness, you should certainly consider it for treating treatment-resistant depression when other drugs have failed.

▶ **Excited schizoaffective patients respond** ◀ **less well to lithium than manics.**

Excited schizoaffective patients respond less well to lithium than do manics; however, some do excellently with lithium. Other schizophrenics do not respond to lithium at all.

Lithium has also been tried experimentally in
- Premenstrual syndrome (if affective symptoms present).
- Emotionally unstable character disorders.
- Periodic psychoses.
- Prevention of schizoaffective episodes.
- Personality disorder with intermittent aggression.

Side Effects and Toxicity

Lithium is not a sedative, and its emotional and intellectual side effects are rare (Table 4.10).

Early Side Effects

These early side effects are common and usually subside in several days.
- Gastrointestinal: nausea, vomiting, diarrhea, stomach pain, taking with meals may help.
- Fatigue, muscle weakness, a dazed feeling.
- Hand tremor which is not affected by AP drugs, but may be controlled by propranolol, a β-adrenergic blocking agent.
- Thirst and frequent urination.

Table 4.10
Lithium Side Effects

Degree	Symptoms
Very mild	Nausea (particularly during first few days of treatment)
	Fine tremor of hands
Mild to moderate	Anorexia
	Vomiting
	Diarrhea
	"Upset stomach" or "abdominal pain"
	Thirst and/or polyuria
	Muscular weakness
	Muscle hyperirritability with twitching, muscle fasciculation or chronic movements
	Sedation, sluggishness, languidness, drowsiness, giddiness
	Coarse tremor
	Ataxia
Moderate to severe	Hypertonic muscles
	Hyperactive deep tendon reflexes
	Hyperextension of arms and legs with grunts and gasping
	Chorea, athetotic movements
	Impairment of consciousness
	Somnolence, confusion, stupor
	Seizures
	Transient focal neurologic signs
	Dysarthria
	Cranial nerve signs
Very severe	Coma
	Complications of coma
	Death

Late Side Effects

- More severe hand tremor
- Polyuria and polydipsia which can be severe; renal diabetes insipidus syndrome, i.e., not affected by vasopressor, but is reversible. May be reversed by careful use of a thiazide diuretic.
- Weight gain and edema
- Nontoxic goiter: this rare side effect is usually mild and can be reduced by thyroxine.
- Latent hypothyroidism can be exacerbated by lithium.
- Possible long-term kidney lesions (interstitial nephritis).

Poisoning

In addition to deliberate overdose, sodium or fluid loss or inter-current illness can cause lithium poisoning.

Early signs, usually present for several days, constitute reasons for stopping lithium and performing a blood test. They include

- Slurred speech
- Drowsiness
- Muscle weakness
- Coarse tremor and muscular twitching
- Dysarthria
- Reappearance of anorexia
- Vomiting and diarrhea
- Ataxia
- Confusion
- Dystonic movements

Late signs of lithium poisoning are predominantly neurologic and include

- Impaired consciousness
- Fasciculation
- Increased deep tendon reflexes
- Attacks of increased muscle tone with hyperextension of arms and legs

This late-poisoning condition is managed by osmotic diuresis (urea), sodium bicarbonate, aminophylline and by dialysis. The latter should be used if significant toxicity is predicted.

Some patients may develop confusion at normal acute lithium blood levels (e.g., 1.5 mEq/liter) and will achieve good therapeutic results with lower dosage and blood levels. This is particularly true in the aged patient.

Leukocytosis (usually about 15,000/mm^3) from a rise in neutro-phils is frequent throughout lithium therapy. ECG changes with T wave depression and widening of the QRS often occur. Rarely, disturbances of the sinus node can occur in those with previously abnormal hearts. Lithium can worsen "sick sinus" syndrome.

Chronic toxicity is particularly troublesome in the elderly patient on maintenance therapy who gradually develops confusion that is falsely attributed to old age. Watch for confusion as a sign of lithium toxicity.

Often you can manage mild lithium toxicity by omitting several doses to allow blood lithium levels to fall, followed by administration of a lower dose.

Lithium can be used safely with antipsychotic agents, or with tricyclic or MAOI antidepressants.

In Pregnancy

Lithium crosses the placental membrane. At the present time it has neither been proven that lithium is safe in pregnancy, nor that lithium is dangerous in pregnancy in humans. Cardiac anomalies have been reported in mothers receiving lithium; however, there is a greater likelihood of such a report being made to a registry when there is an anomaly than a report being made when the child is normal. In prospective studies, no differences were noted. However, the number of lithium pregnancies are too small to rule out a teratogenic effect. Because of lithium's potential danger, it is not recommended unless there is a severe clinical need for it. Lithium does appear in breast milk.

SUMMARY: THE POWER OF PSYCHOACTIVE DRUGS

A meaningful quantitative number is the empirically measured drug-placebo difference for overall efficacy for a specific drug administered to patients with a given disease. For example, the drug-placebo difference of imipramine to treat acute depression can be calculated. There are essentially 30 double-blind comparisons of imipramine vs. placebo in treating depression. From this data we dichotomize the patients who did (relatively) well, having a substantial improvement or recovery, as well as the patient who did not do well in both the drug group and in the placebo group. The results of this calculation are presented in Table 4.11 showing a highly significant drug-placebo difference using the method of Fleiss. These results can also be expressed as a percentage of patients who do well or not well on drug and placebo, or as a phi coefficient. This is essentially a product-moment correlation coefficient for dichotomy data, the higher the correlation, the bigger the drug-placebo difference. In Chapter 3, on Antipsychotic Drugs, we present a comparison of antipsychotics for acute schizophrenia as well as streptomycin for tuberculosis. The data from this figure (3.5) were dichotomized and are presented in Table 4.12 as an overall comparison of drug efficacy. Also, in Chapter 3, we presented data on 29 studies of antipsychotics for a prophylaxis against future relapses of schizophrenia. The number of subjects

Table 4.11
Effectiveness of Tricyclic Antidepressants*

Imipramine	65%
Placebo	32%

R = .32 $p = 1 \times 10^{-31}$

* Results of 30 double-blind studies of 1334 patients. Percentage of patients greatly improved or recovered at 3–4 weeks.

Table 4.12
Percentage of Patients Who Do Well on Various Treatments

		Well	Poor	R
Antipsychotic for treatment of acute schizophrenia	Drug	70%	25%	.45
	Placebo	30%	75%	
Maintenance antipsychotic for prophylaxis	Drug	80%	20%	.34
	Placebo	47%	53%	
Imipramine acute depression	Drug	65%	35%	.33
	Placebo	32%	68%	
Tricyclic prophylaxis of depression	Drug	73%	27%	.26
	Placebo	48%	52%	
Lithium acute mania	Drug	73%	28%	.38
	Placebo	34%	66%	
Lithium prophylaxis of mania depression	Drug	63%	37%	.43
	Placebo	21%	79%	
Streptomycin for tuberculosis	Drug	69%	33%	.36
	Standard	31%	67%	
Penicillin for pneumococcal pneumonia	Penicillin	93%	6%	.10
	Sulfanilamide	88%	11%	
Drugs in surgery—1964–72	New	63%	37%	.06
	Old	57%	43%	

having relapses or doing well was summated from data in this table and is presented in Table 4.12 as the overall efficacy comparison of maintenance for prophylaxis. Similarly, in this chapter there are data on tricyclic prophylaxis of depression or lithium prophylaxis for both bipolar and unipolar disorders and again this data is summated and presented here. Similar data collected by Peter Stokes are available for the lithium treatment of acute mania. The classic antibiotics are streptomycin for tuberculosis and penicillin for pneumococcal pneumonia. When penicillin was initially used for pneumococcal pneumonia, sulfanilamide was the standard drug. Note that the penicillin was a substantially better drug than sulfanilamide. Indeed, the death rate from pneumonia for patients receiving sulfanilamide was essentially double the rate observed when they received penicillin. The miracles of streptomycin and penicillin are not typical of average medical advances. To measure the everyday medical advances, as opposed to the major breakthroughs, we identified all of the controlled studies which used drugs in a new way in surgery in comparison to the standard treatments. This was based on studies published between 1964 and 1972. The average improvement in patients who do well is a 6% increment, from 57% to 63%. This is, of course, an average of many innovations. Some produced improvement. In others the patients did about the same on the new treatment *vs.* the old treatment. For some innovations, the patients did better on the old treatment. It would seem that in terms of the drug-placebo difference, the improvement with the psychotropic drugs is comparable to major innovations in chemotherapy. Indeed, the discovery of effective psychotropic drugs is as much a breakthrough for psychiatry as the discovery of antibiotics was a breakthrough for medicine. We would caution against an over-concrete interpretation of such data. There is no way a quantitative comparison can be made on efficacy of drugs for different disorders. We do feel, however, that a quantitation of the drug-placebo difference allows a convenient way to express drug-placebo differences. Namely, the expression of drug placebo difference in a four-fold table provides an easy way to quantitate the drug-placebo difference, allowing the reader to intuitively make a qualitative comparison between drug efficacy for one disease vs. another. You cannot make a quantitative comparison here because the disorders are qualitatively different. The value for having such a table is that you can look at the drug placebo difference, holding in your mind the qualitative difference between the diseases treated and drug effects. The purpose of this table is to give the reader some quantitative data to facilitate qualitative comparisons.

References

Plasma Tricyclics

Asberg, M., Cromholm, B., Sjoquist, F., et al.: Relationship between plasma levels and therapeutic effect of nortriptyline. Br. Med. J. 3:331, 1971.

Biggs, J. T., and Zeigler, V. E.: Protriptyline plasma levels and antidepressant response. Clin. Pharmacol. Ther. 22:269–273, 1978.

Braithwaite, R. A., Goulding, R., Theano, G., et al.: Plasma concentration of amitriptyline and clinical response. Lancet 1: 1297, 1972.

Glassman, A. H., and Perel, J. M.: Plasma levels and tricyclic antidepressants. Clin. Pharmacol. Ther. *16:* 198–200, 1974. Part 2.

Glassman, A. H., Perel, J. M., Shostak, M., *et al.*: Clinical implications of imipramine plasma levels for depressive illness. Arch. Gen. Psychiatric 34:197–204, 1977.

Kragh-Sorenson, P., Asberg, M., and Eggert-Hansen, C.: Plasma nortriptyline levels in endogenous depression. Lancet *1*:113, 1973.

Kragh-Sorensen, P., Eggert-Hansen, C., Banstrup, P. C., *et al.*: Self-inhibiting action of nortriptyline antidepressive effect at high plasma levels. Psychopharmacologia *45*:305–312, 1976a.

Kragh-Sorensen, P., Hansen, L. E., and Asberg, M.: Plasma levels of nortriptyline in the treatment of endogenous depression. Acta Psychiatr. Scand. *49:* 445–456, 1973.

Kupfer, D. J., Hanin, I., Spiker, D. G., *et al.*: Amitriptyline plasma levels and clinical response in primary depression. Clin. Pharmacol. Ther. 22:904–911, 1977.

Montgomery, S. A., Braithwaite, R. A., and Crammer, J. L.: Routine nortriptyline levels in treatment of depression. Br. Med. J. 2:166–167, 1977.

Montgomery, S., Braithwaite, R., Dawling, S., *et al.*: High plasma nortriptyline levels in the treatment of depression, I. Clin. Pharmacol. Ther. 23:309–314, 1978.

Muscettola, G., Goodwin, F. K., Potter, W. Z., *et al.*: Imipramine and desipramine in plasma and spinal fluid. Arch. Gen. Psychiatry 35:621–625, 1978.

Olivier-Martin, R., Marzin, D., Buschenschutz, E., *et al.*: Concentrations plasmatiques de l'imipramine et de la desmethylimipramine et effet antidepresseur au cours d'un traitement controle. Psychopharmacologia *41:* 187–195, 1975.

Reisby, N., Gram, L. F., Bach, P., *et al.*: Imipramine: Clinical effects and pharmacokinetic variability. Psychopharmacology 54:263–272, 1977.

Whyte, S. F., MacDonald, A. J., Naylor, G. J., *et al.*: Plasma concentrations of protriptyline and clinical effects in depressed women. Br. J. Psychiatry 128:394–390, 1976.

Zeigler, V. E., Clayton, P. J., and Biggs, J. T.: A comparison study of amitriptyline and nortriptyline with plasma levels. Arch. Gen. Psychiatry 34:607–612, 1977.

Maintenance Antidepressants

Baastrup, P. C., Poulsen, J. C., Schou, M., *et al.*: Prophylactic lithium: double-blind discontinuation in manic-depressive and recurrent depressive disorders. Lancet *1*:326–330, 1970.

Coppen, A., Noguera, R., and Bailey, J.: Prophylactic lithium in affective disorder. Lancet 2:275–279, 1971.

Coppen, A., Ghose, K., Montgomery, S., *et al.*: Continuation therapy with amitriptyline in depression. Br. J. Psychiatry 133:28–33, 1978.

Cundall, R. L., Brooks, P. W., and Murray, L. S.: A controlled evaluation of lithium prophylaxis in affective disorders. Psychol. Med. 2:308–311, 1972.

Fieve, R., Kumbaraci, T., and Dunner, D. L.: Lithium prophylaxis of depression in bipolar I, bipolar II and unipolar patients. Am. J. Psychiatry *133:* 925–929, 1978.

Fieve, R., Dunner, D. L., Kumbaraci, T., *et al.*: Lithium carbonate prophylaxis of depression in three subtypes of primary affective disorders. Pharmacopsychiatry 9:100–107, 1976.

Hullen, R., McDonald, R., and Allsopp, M.: Prophylactic lithium in recurrent affective disorders. Lancet 1:1044–1046, 1972.

Kay, D. W. K.., Fahy, T., and Garside, R. F.: A seven-month double blind trial of amitriptyline and diazepam in ECT-treated depressed patients. Br. J. Psychiatry 117:667, 1970.

Klerman, G. L., DiMascio, A., Weisman, M., *et al.*: Treatment of depression by drugs and psychotherapy. Am. J. Psychiatry 131:186–191, 1974.

Melia, P. I.: Prophylactic lithium: a double-blind trial in recurrent affective disorders. Br. J. Psychiatry 116:621–624, 1970.

Mindham, R. H. S., Howland, D., and Shepard, M.: An evaluation of continuation therapy with tricyclic antidepressants in depressive illness. Psychol. Med. 3:5-17, 1973.

Mindham, R. H. S., Howland, C., and Shepherd, M.: Continuation therapy with tricyclic antidepressants in depressive illness. Lancet 2:854, 1972.

Persson, G.: Lithium prophylaxis in affective disorders. Acta Psychiatry Scand. 48:462-479, 1972.

Prien, R., Caffey, E., and Klett, C. J.: Prophylactic efficacy of lithium carbonate in manic depressive illness. Arch. Gen. Psychiatry 28:337-341, 1973.

Prien, R. F., Caffey, E. M., Jr., and Klett, C. J.: Lithium carbonate and imipramine in prevention of affective episodes. Arch. Gen. Psychiatry 29:420-425, 1973.

Quitkin, F., Rifkin, A., Kane, J., et al.: Prophylactic effect of lithium and imipramine in unipolar and bipolar II patients. Am. J. Psychiatry 135:570-572, 1978.

Seager, C. P., and Bird, R. L.: Imipramine with electrical treatment in depression controlled trial. J. Ment. Sci. 108: 704, 1962.

Sheehy, L. M., and Maxmen, J.: Phenelzine induced psychosis: Am. J. Psychiatry 135:1422-3, 1978.

Monoamine Oxidase Inhibitors

Agnew, P. C., Baran, I. D., Klapman, H. J. et al.: A clinical evaluation of four antidepressant drugs (Nardil, Tofranil, Marplan and Deprol). Am. J. Psychiatry 118:160-162, 1961.

Clinical Psychiatry Committee of the Medical Research Council. Clinical trial of the treatment of depressive illness. Br. Med. J. 1:881, 1965.

Greenblatt, M., Grosser, G. H., and Wechsler, H.: Differential response of hospitalized depressed patients to somatic therapy. Am. J. Psychiatry 120: 935-943, 1964.

Hare, E. H., Dominian, J., and Sharpe, L.: Phenelzine and dexamphetamine in depressive illness: A comparative trial. Br. Med. J. 5270:9-12, 1962.

Johnstone, E. C., and Marsh, W.: Acetylator status and response to phenelzine in depressed patients. Lancet 1: 567-570, 1973.

Lascalles, R. G.: Atypical facial pain and depression. Br. J. Psychiatry 112:651-659, 1966.

Raskin, A., Schulterbrandt, J. G., Reatig, N., et al.: Depression subtypes and response to phenelzine, diazepam and a placebo. Arch. Gen. Psychiatry 30:66-75, 1974.

Ravaris, C. L., Nies, A., Robinson, D. S., et al.: A multiple-dose, controlled study of phenelzine in depression-anxiety states. Arch. Gen. Psychiatry 33:347-350, 1976.

Rees, L., and Davis, B. A controlled trial of phenelzine (Nardil) in the treatment of severe depressive illness. J. Ment. Sci. 107:560-566, 1961.

Robinson, D., Nies, A., Ravaris, C. L., et al.: Clinical pharmacology of phenelzine. Arch. Gen. Psychiatry 35:629-635, 1978.

Robinson, D. S., Nies, A., Ravaris, C. L., et al.: The monoamine oxidase inhibitor, phenelzine, in the treatment of depressive-anxiety states. Arch. Gen. Psychiatry 29:407-413, 1973.

Schildkraut, J. J., Klerman, G. L., Hammond, R., et al.: Excretion of 3-methoxy-4-hydroxy-mandelic acid (VMA) in depressed patients treated with antidepressant drugs. J. Psychiatr. Res. 2:257-266, 1965.

General

Bigger, J. T., Jr., Giardina, E. G. V., Perel, J. M., et al.: Cardiac antiarrhythmic effect of imipramine hydrochloride. N. Engl. J. Med. 296:206-208, 1977.

Blackwell, B., Stefopoulos, A., Enders, P., et al.: Anticholinergic activity of two tricyclic antidepressants. Am. J. Psychiatry 135:722-724, 1978.

Bunney, W. E., Jr., and Davis, J. M.: Norepinephrine in depressive reactions. Arch. Gen. Psychiatry 13:483, 1965.

Coryell, W.: Intrapatient response to ECT and tricyclic antidepressants. Am. J. Psychiatry 135:1108-10, 1978.

Covi, L., Lipman, R. S., Derogatis, L. R.,

et al.: Drugs and group psychotherapy in neurotic depression. Am. J. Psychiatry 131:191–198, 1974.

Chane, G. E.: Iproniazid (Marsalid) phosphate, a therapeutic agent for mental disorders and debilitating disease. Psychiatr. Res. Rep. 8:142–152, 1957.

Davis, J. M., Bartlett, E., and Termini, B. A.: Overdosage of psychotropic drugs. Dis. Nerv. Syst. 29:157, 246, 1968.

Davis, J. M., Klerman, G. L., and Schildkraut, J. J.: Drugs used in the treatment of depression. In *Psychopharmacology: A Review of Progress, 1957–1967,* p. 625. Washington, D.C., U. S. Government Printing Office, 1968.

Dysken, M. W., Evans, H. M., Chan, C. H., *et al.*: Improvement of depression and parkinsonism during ECT: a case study. Neuropsychobiology 2:81–86, 1976.

Everett, H.: The use of betanechol chloride with tricyclic antidepressants. Am. J. Psychiatry 132:1202–4, 1975.

Fann, W. E., Cavanaugh, J. H., Kaufmann, J. S., *et al.*: Doxepin: Effects on transport of biogenic amines. Psychopharmacologia 22:111–125, 1971.

Gelenberg, A. J., and Klerman, G. L.: Antidepressants: Their use in clinical practice. Rational Drug Ther. 12:1–7, April, 1978.

Glassman, A., Kantor, S., and Shostak, M.: Depression, delusions, and drug response. Am. J. Psychiatry 132:716–719, 1975.

Hollister, L. E.: Tricyclic antidepressants. N. Engl. J. Med. 299:1106–9, 1168–72, 1978.

Fann, W. E., Janowsky, D. S., Oates, J. A., *et al.*: Chlorpromazine reversal of the antihypertensive action of guanethidine. Lancet 2:436, 1971.

Fawcett, J., Maas, J. W., and Dekirmenjian, H.: Depression and MHPG excretion response to dextroamphetamine and tricyclic antidepressants. Arch. Gen. Psychiatry 26:246, 1972.

Fink, M., Klein, D. F., and Kramer, J. C.: Clinical efficacy of chlorpromazine-procyclidine combination, impramine, and placebo in depressive disorders. Psychopharmacologia 7:27, 1965.

Finnerty, R., Goldberg, H. L., and Rickels, K.: Doxepin versus imipramine in psychoneurotic depressed patients with sleep disturbance. J. Clin. Psychiatry 39:852–56, 1978.

Fleiss, J. L.: *Statistical Methods for Rates and Proportions.* New York, John Wiley & Sons, 1973.

Horden, A., Burt, C. G., and Holt, N. F.: *Depressive States.* Springfield, Ill., Charles C Thomas, 1965.

Johnstone, E. C.: The relationship between acetylator status and inhibitor of monoamine oxidase, excretion of free drug and antidepressant response in depressed patients on phenelzine. Psychopharmacologia 46: 289–294, 1976.

Kiloh, L. G., Ball, J. R. B., and Garside, R. F.: Prognostic factors in treatment of depressive states with imipramine. Br. Med. J. 1:1225, 1962.

Klein, D. F.: Importance of psychiatric diagnosis in prediction of clinical drug effects. Arch. Gen. Psychiatry 16:1188–1926, 1967.

Klein, D. F., and Davis, J. M.: *Diagnosis and Drug Treatment of Psychiatric Disorders.* Baltimore, Williams & Wilkins, 1969.

Klerman, G. L., and Cole, J. O.: Clinical pharmacology of imipramine and related antidepressants compounds. Pharmacol. Rev. 17:101, 1965.

Klerman, G. L. and Hirschfeld, R.: The use of antidepressants in clinical practice. J.A.M.A. 240:1403–6, 1978.

Kuhn, R.: The treatment of depressive states with G#22355 (imipramine hydrochloride). Am. J. Psychiatry 115: 459, 1958.

Loomer, H. P., Saunders, J. C., and Kline, N. S.: A clinical and pharmacodynamic evaluation of iproniazid as a psychic energizer. Psychiatr. Res. Rep. 8:129, 1957.

Maas, J. W.: Biogenic amines and depression: Biochemical and pharmacological separation of two types of depression. Arch. Gen. Psychiatry 32: 1357–1361, 1975.

Maas, J. W., Fawcett, J. A., and Dekirmenjian, H.: 3-methoxy-4-hydroxy phenylglycol (MHPG) excretion in depressive states. Arch. Gen. Psychiatry 19:129, 1968.

MacLean, R., Nicholson, W. J., Pare, C. M. B., et al.: Effect of monoamine oxidase inhibitors on the concentration of 5-hydroxytryptamine in the human brain. Lancet 2:205–208, 1965.

Moir, D. C., Crooks, J., Sawyer, P., et al.: Cardiotoxicity of tricyclic antidepressants. Br. J. Pharmacol. 44:371, 1972.

Murphy, D. L.: The behavioral toxicity of monoamine oxidase inhibiting antidepressants. Adv. Pharmacol. Chemother. 14:71–105, 1977.

Pare, C. M. B., Rees, L., and Sainsbury, M. J.: Differentiation of two genetically specific types of depression by the response to antidepressants. Lancet 2:1340, 1962.

Paykel, E. S., Parker, R. R., Penrose, R., et al.: Prediction of phenenzine outcome in depressive. Neuropharmacology 17:105–7, 1978.

Peterson, G., Blackwell, B., Hostetler, R., et al.: Anticholinergic activity of the tricyclic antidepressants desipramine and doxepin in nondepressed volunteers. Commun. Psychopharmacol. 2: 145–150, 1978.

Quitkin, F. M., Rifkin, A., Kaplan, J., Klein, D. F., and Oaks, G.: Phobic anxiety syndrome complicated by drug dependence and addiction. Arch. Gen. Psychiatry 27:159, 1972.

Quitkin, F., Rifkin, A., and Klein, D. F.: Imipramine response in deluded depressive patients. Am. J. Psychiatry 135:806–811, 1978.

Sandifer, M. G., Wilson, I. C., and Gambill, J. M.: The influence of case selection and dosage in antidepressant drug trial. Br. J. Psychiatry 111:142, 1965.

Sargant, W.: Drugs in the treatment of depression. Br. Med. J. 1:225–227, 1961.

Schildkraut, J. J.: The catecholamine hypothesis of affective disorder. A review of supporting evidence. Am. J. Psychiatry 122:509, 1965.

Simpson, G., Amin, M., Angus, J., et al.: Role of antidepressants and neuroleptics in the treatment of depression. Arch. Gen. Psychiatry 27:337–345, 1972.

Simpson, G. M., Lee, J. H., Cuculic, Z., et al.: Two dosages of imipramine in hospitalized endogenous and neurotic depressives. Arch. Gen. Psychiatry 33:1093–1102, 1976.

Snyder, S. H., and Yamamura, H. I.: Antidepressants and the muscarinic acetylcholine receptor. Arch. Gen. Psychiatry 31:236–239, 1977.

Squire, L. P., and Chace, P. M.: Memory function six to nine months after electroconvulsive therapy. Arch. Gen. Psychiatry 32:1557–1564, 1975.

Suiser, F., Vetulani, J., and Mooley, P.: Mode of action of antidepressant drugs. Biochem. Pharmacol. 27:257–261, 1978.

Sweeney, D., and Maas, J.: Specificity of depressive disease. Ann. Rev. Med. 29:219–29, 1978.

Uhlenhuth, E. H., and Park, L. C.: The influence of medication imipramine and doctor in relieving depressed psychoneurotic outpatients. J. Psychiatr. Res. 2:101, 1964.

Wilson, I. C., Vernon, J. T., Guin, T., et al.: A controlled study of treatments of depression. J. Neuropsychiatry 4: 331, 1963.

Wittenborn, J. R., Plante, M., Burgess, F., et al.: Comparison of imipramine, electroconvulsive therapy and placebo in the treatment of depression. J. Nerv. Ment. Dis. 135:131, 1962.

chapter FIVE

Antianxiety Agents: Adjunct to Psychotherapy

DIAGNOSING NEUROSES AND PERSONALITY DISORDERS

The psychoneurotic states are characterized by anxiety and the absence of gross distortion of reality or personality disorganization. The patient uses defense mechanisms to diminish anxiety, and these defenses give rise to the specific psychoneurotic subtypes:
- Anxiety reaction.
- Dissociative reaction.
- Conversion reaction.
- Phobic reaction.
- Obsessive compulsive reaction.

A neurotic may experience severe anxiety while not having the defenses to cope with even moderate amounts. Mistrusting his own competence and interpreting his environment as potentially hostile, he attempts to avoid psychological pain. He is denied the hearty and spontaneous experiences of life, and his reality contact and capacity to communicate emotions are restricted. Confronted with a new anxiety-producing situation, he cannot overcome the challenge and grow, but becomes paralyzed by his own fear.

Anxiety is classified into two main types: *panic anxiety* that results in feeling suddenly overwhelmed by fearful sensations flooding a seemingly helpless personality; and *anticipatory (signal) anxiety*, a less intense fear resulting from assessing a situation as potentially overwhelming and panic-producing. This anxiety acts as a signal of what might happen.

Each patient experiences anxiety in his own way. Various somatic patterns include cardiovascular, gastrointestinal, urinary, respiratory and musculoskeletal symptoms.

In personality or character disorders, the conflict becomes latent. Instead of producing painful neurotic symptoms, the ego is permanently altered and rigid defense attitudes are prominent.

The primary treatment for the neurotic is psychotherapy. Drugs can occasionally be useful and when properly employed augment psychotherapy. The relationship between antianxiety agents and interpersonal treatment has been explored in a few controlled studies. The evidence clearly suggests that pharmacotherapy in no way interferes with psychotherapy.

The Diagnostic and Statistical Manual of the American Psychiatric Association (DSM III) has done away with the neurosis as a diagnosis category, but in a somewhat broader sense we will on occasion use the term "neurotic" to refer to a larger category of mental disease, including anxiety disorders, somatoform disorders, and dissociative disorders. Below is a classification of the "neurotic" and personality disorders. Note that the schizophrenia-like personality disorders such as paranoid, schizoid, schizotypal and borderline personality disorders is discussed in our section on Schizophrenia.

Anxiety Disorders

Phobic disorder (Phobic neurosis)
   Agoraphobia with panic attacks
   Agoraphobia without panic attacks
   Social phobia
   Simple phobia
Anxiety state (Anxiety neurosis)
   Panic disorder
   Generalized anxiety disorder
   Obsessive compulsive disorder
   (Obsessive compulsive neurosis)
Post-traumatic stress disorder
   Acute
   Chronic or delayed
   Atypical anxiety disorder

Somatoform Disorders

Somatization disorder
Conversion disorder
(Hysterical neurosis, conversion type)
Psychogenic pain disorder
Hypochondriasis
(Hypochondriacal neurosis)
Atypical somatoform disorder

Dissociative Disorders (Hysterical Neuroses, Dissociative Type)

Psychogenic amnesia
Psychogenic fugue
Multiple personality
Depersonalization disorder
(Depersonalization neurosis)
Atypical dissociative disorder

Personality Disorders

Paranoid
Schizoid
Schizotypal

Histrionic
Narcissistic
Antisocial
Borderline

Avoidant
Dependent
Compulsive
Passive-Aggressive

Typical diagnostic criteria for some of the anxiety disorders are listed below:

Agoraphobia

A. The individual avoids being alone where he cannot get to help, or help cannot get to him, in case of sudden incapacitation.
B. These fears are pervasive and dominate the patients life so that a large number of situations are entered into only reluctantly or are avoided. The individual avoids at least one of the following situations:

    (1) Closed or open spaces.
    (2) Traveling while alone.
    (3) Traveling more than five miles from home by any means.
    (4) Walking alone.
    (5) Being alone.
C. Marked anxiety is experienced when faced with the potential of being in one of the above situations.
D. The phobic symptoms are not symptomatic of an episode of Major Depressive Disorder, Obsessive Compulsive Disorder, or Schizophrenia.

Social Phobia

A. Avoidance of an irrationally feared specific social situation with overconcern about humiliation and embarrassment.
B. Avoidance behavior (actual avoidance or compelling desire to avoid phobic stimulus) is a significant source of distress or interferes with social or role functioning.
C. The patient recognizes the irrational nature of his fear.
D. The avoidance is not symptomatic of another mental disorder, such as Obsessive Compulsive Disorder or Schizophrenia.

Simple Phobia

A. Avoidance of the irrationally feared object or situation. If there is any element of danger in these objects or situations, it is reacted to out of proportion to reality.
B. Avoidance behavior (actual avoidance or compelling desire to avoid phobic stimulus) is a significant source of distress or interferes with social or role functioning.
C. The patient recognizes the irrational nature of his fear.
D. The phobic symptoms are not symptomatic of another mental disorder, such as Obsessive Compulsive Disorder or Schizophrenia.

Panic Disorder

A. At least three panic attacks, occurring within a three week period and occurring at times other than during marked physical exertion or a life-threatening situation, and in the absence of a physical disorder that could account for the symptoms of the anxiety. Further, these attacks do not occur only upon exposure to a circumscribed phobic stimulus.

B. The panic attacks are manifested by discrete periods of apprehension or fearfulness, with at least four of the following symptoms present during the majority of attacks:
   (1) Dyspnea.
   (2) Palpitations.
   (3) Chest pain or discomfort.
   (4) Choking or smothering sensations.
   (5) Dizziness, vertigo or unsteady feelings.
   (6) Feelings of unreality.
   (7) Paresthesias.
   (8) Hot and cold flashes.
   (9) Sweating.
   (10) Faintness.
   (11) Trembling or shaking.
   (12) Fear of dying, going crazy or doing something uncontrolled during an attack.
C. The panic attacks are not symptomatic of another mental disorder.
D. Not meet the criteria for Agoraphobia.

Generalized Anxiety Disorder

A. Generalized and persistent anxiety manifested by symptoms from three of the four categories noted in the essential features: motor tension, autonomic hyperactivity, apprehensive expectation, vigilance and scanning.
B. The anxious mood has lasted continuously for at least six months.
C. The onset is not associated with a psychosocial stressor.
D. The disturbance is not symptomatic of another mental disorder, such as Depressive Disorders or Schizophrenia.
E. Age at least 18.

Obsessive Compulsive Disorder

A. Obsessions and/or compulsions. Obsessions are recurrent, persistent ideas, thoughts, images or impulses which are ego-alien. Compulsions are behaviors that are not experienced as the outcome of the individual's own volition, but are accompanied by a sense of subjective compulsion and a desire to resist (at least initially).
B. The patient recognizes the senselessness of the behavior.

C. The obsessions or compulsions are a significant source of distress to the individual or interfere with social or role functioning.
D. The obsessions or compulsions are not symptomatic of Major Depressive Disorder, Schizophrenia, or Organic Mental Disorder.

WHEN TO USE AN ANTIANXIETY AGENT (AA)

General Characteristics of AAs (Minor Tranquilizers)

AAs are more like sedative-hypnotic drugs such as barbiturates, than like major tranquilizers, such as the phenothiazines. As with barbiturates, high-dose AAs can produce delirium, nervousness, convulsions and insomnia upon sudden withdrawal. The convulsions can occur up to two weeks after withdrawal of either drug. Easily addicted patients tend to abuse both drug groups.

AAs have no antipsychotic effect and do not produce extrapyramidal side effects. This defines the group and sharply distinguishes it from the antipsychotic agents. They have anticonvulsant and muscle relaxant properties.

Sedative Capabilities

The margin between anxiety relief and sedation is much wider with AAs than with the barbituates.

► **Warn patients about drinking while taking AAs.** ◄

The sedative effect, which can initially impair performance, is also potentiated by alcohol and central nervous system depressants. Patients should be warned about drinking.

Tolerance

In some patients, the therapeutic effect wanes after three or four weeks. Possible causes are placebo relief of a chronic state, or metabolic or tissue tolerance.

Occasionally, the patient voluntarily, and without notifying the physician, increases the dosage to regain the initial euphoric effect. Barbiturates have a greater liability for abuse than AAs. Indeed, a further difference between an AA and an antipsychotic agent is the AA's euphoric effect. Patients get no pleasure from antipsychotics and never voluntarily increase their dosage.

Suicide with AAs is difficult (except for meprobamate). This makes them desirable for patients who are upset and whose behavior is potentially self-destructive.

Target Symptoms Responsive to AAs

The results of treating anxiety cannot be judged solely by symptomatic relief. Just because subjective distress subsides does *not* mean there is improvement if it is accompanied by growth avoidance, productivity loss and absence of interpersonal relationships. Nevertheless, the outstanding indication for AA use is anticipatory anxiety.

AAs are most useful in acute, anxious, reactive, anticipatory situations, but acute patients improve on anything, so that the drug-placebo difference is difficult or impossible to show. AAs do have a significant edge over barbiturates and placebos in chronic anxiety states. To avoid life-long use, you must eliminate the cause of the anxiety or increase the patient's tolerance for it. Dangers of AA use include tolerance, ever-increasing dosage, psychological dependence and addiction.

Other Uses and Indications for AAs

- Psychosomatic disorders with anxiety
- Restlessness, agitation, insomnia, tension and excitability
- Senile agitation
- Acute alcoholism
- Muscle disorders
- Convulsive disorders

Which Neurotic Patients Benefit from AAs?

Anxiety Disorders

AAs are effective for treating anxiety reactions, but are often unnecessary in acute states, which tend to remit promptly without drugs. Prescribe an AA only if the distress is severe.

One primary use of AAs is for treating simple anxiety reactions. When distress is severe, crippling and constricting, symptomatic relief with AAs can facilitate psychotherapy, new learning and coping with reality problems. Situations may exist where you will not wish to remove the symptoms with drugs. For example, if one expected the symptoms to subside because of changes in the patient's life, it would not be desirable to cloud the situation with a drug effect. Anti-anxiety medication is only one of several therapeutic techniques you can use after carefully evaluating the patient's problems.

Dissociative and Somatoform Disorders

AAs are *not* effective with conversion reactions. Hyteroschizophrenics have rapidly fluctuating psychoses and are *indifferent* to their delusions. Believing and proclaiming that their food is poisoned, they will nevertheless eat it. A schizophrenic will not. Drug treatment has generally been disappointing for dissociative and somatoform disorders; useful mainly to treat anxiety as it overtly occurs in the patient.

Phobic Disorders

AAs are moderately effective against anxiety, but the phobia remains. With phobic anxiety, patients experience separation anxiety, panic attacks and travel phobia. Antidepressants stop the panic attacks, but not the anticipatory anxiety. The patient continues to expect the attacks and does not realize that the panic will diminish or disappear if the dreaded event actually occurs. So he may insist that there is no improvement. AAs diminish the anticipatory anxiety and the patient generally feels better.

Klein has described this syndrome which is characterized by severe panic attacks, i.e., sudden, spontaneous, unexpected feelings of terror and anxiety, plus the autonomic equivalence of anxiety and the desire to flee and return to a safe place. The diagnostic criteria are listed in Table 5.1. The patient may well have two disorders, the panic attacks and the fear of places where these attacks occur. As a result of having panic attacks, the patients then began to show anticipatory anxiety. The Hillside group verified that the panic attack gradually is helped by imipramine, but also showed that simple phobias are not helped. The primary

Table 5.1
Phobic Anxiety Syndrome

1. Sudden spontaneous unexplained panic attack characterized by feeling of terror, autonomic symptoms of anxiety and a flight response
2. Symptoms during an attack can be
   a. anxiety, terror, helpless, impending doom
   b. smothering or choking feeling, difficulty getting breath
      dizzy or faint
      trembling
      tingling, hot or cold spells
      chest pain or discomfort
      nausea
      palpitation and rapid heart beat
      sudden empty feeling in pit of stomach
3. Fear of places where attacks occur
   a. Public places (restaurants, stores, buses, etc.)
   b. Fear that cannot reach secure place such as home

symptom is the panic attack itself. The fear of places where such attacks have occurred, or might possibly occur, is a secondary elaboration of the symptom.

For this reason, we would prefer to call this a panic attacks syndrome because the "agoraphobia" or "fear of the market place" or fear of public places is a secondary reaction to the panic attacks. These attacks occur when the patient is, in some sense, separated from significant others—traveling alone in subways, tunnels, bridges, or out in the streets. The patient then begins to show anticipatory anxiety and dread of situations that may get him in the situation of which he is phobic. The patients typically have been fearful, dependent children with a great deal of separation anxiety. Imipramine dramatically stops the panic attacks. Psychological treatment is sometimes useful for overcoming the anticipatory anxiety and helping the patient to go back into the situation in which he experienced the panic attack so that he can demonstrate to himself that he no longer experiences it. Imipramine is specific for the panic attack, but does not help the anticipatory anxiety. Its efficacy has been demonstrated in a double blind study. Quitkin et al. (1972) further note that a serious complication of this syndrome is abuse of sedatives and alcohol through self-medication. The patients on imipramine did well and did not return to alcohol or drug abuse, but the control group (not maintained on imipramine) did return to drug abuse, which necessitated rehospitalization. The childhood version of this syndrome (school phobia) is also helped by imipramine. This syndrome of phobic anxiety is, in many respects, a pharmacologically defined syndrome, defined by its prevention by tricyclic antidepressants. In addition, note that phobias are not a specific syndrome, but rather a symptom: e.g., one subtype of childhood psychopathology may be this panic attack syndrome and, hence, treatable with drugs.

At about the same time that Klein was investigating imipramine in the United States, investigators in England noted that some patients with hysteria or secondary depression responded to monoamine oxidase inhibitors (MAOIs). Subsequently, several researchers in England and Canada showed MAOIs to be superior to placebo in hysterics with phobic symptoms, a subcategorization which might be similar to the agoraphobia described by Klein. These results are summarized in Table 5.2 and Table 5.3. We prefer, as a summary table, information on the percentage of patients who do recover, or who show substantial improvement, moderate improvement, minimal improvement, no change or worsening, etc. Unfortunately, some studies only provide mean change scores. (Table 5.3).

Thus, we require two tables to summarize the information. Note that three studies consistently find imipramine effective for agoraphobia, and four studies find MAOIs effective for agoraphobia or phobic anxiety.

There is insufficient evidence to define whether MAO inhibitors or tricyclics are superior in treating the syndrome, but there is an accumulating body of evidence supporting the efficacy of these drugs. That is why we have emphasized the topic by presenting the raw data in tabular form. This allows the reader of the data to arrive at his own judgment. We feel the practicing psychiatrist should watch for the syndrome, and, when it occurs, treat it with tricyclics or MAOIs, as these are agents with proven efficacy. Research will have to determine the cause and which of the two treatments is most effective. (See references on Phobic Anxiety.)

Obsessive-Compulsive Disorders and Compulsive Personality Disorders

These patients do not believe in the reality of the unwanted ideas and ego-alien impulses they feel forced to obey, whereas schizophrenics do. The evidence on drug treatment is limited but

Table 5.2

Effect of Imipramine or Phenelzine in Agoraphobia

| Effect | Percentage of patients improved or not improved | | | | | | |
| | Zitrin et al. study | | Sheehan et al. study | | | Solyom et al. study | |
	Imipramine	Behavioral therapy	Phenelzine	Imipramine	Placebo	Phenelzine	Placebo
Marked	53%	18%	59%	28%	18%	9%	0%
Moderate	42%	54%	35%	61%	32%*	82%	40%
Minimal	2%	21%	—	—	—	—	—
No change	2%	7%	6%	11%	50%	9%	60%
No. of subjects	43	18	17	18	22	11	10
	p = .01		p = .001		p = .025	p = .02	

* Partial improvement.

Table 5.3

Effect of Imipramine or Phenelzine on Agoraphobia or Phobic Anxiety
(Mean improvement on drug or placebo)

	Mean outcome	Anxiety rating	(Overall psychiatrist rating difference 0–8 weeks)
Agoraphobia (Klein)			
Imipramine	6.4		
Placebo	2.0		
N =	19		
P	.001		
Agoraphobia (Lipsedge et al.)			
Phenelzine		2.29	
Placebo		1.60	
N =		59	
P =		.026	
Phobic anxiety (Tyrer et al.)			
Phenelzine			2.18
Placebo			.75
N =			28
P =			.026

several studies suggest that chlorimipramine and/or tryptophan may be effective.

Mixed Anxiety Depression

No official American Psychiatric Association diagnosis exists for patients exhibiting mixed anxiety and depression. They sometimes are diagnosed as having an anxiety reaction or, at other times, as experiencing a psychoneurotic depression. Many agents are used to treat this condition: antipsychotics, tricyclic antidepressants, minor tranquilizers, a combination of phenothiazines and tricyclic antidepressants or MAOIs.

Doxepin is said to possess antianxiety properties similar to minor tranquilizers, as well as antidepressant properties similar to the TCAs. Controlled studies indicate that doxepin is effective for mixed anxiety and depression in outpatients (Table 5.4). Tricyclic antidepressants and minor tranquilizers alone are both effective in treating mixed anxiety-depression syndromes. Because this is a heterogenous population, antidepressants may help those who are depressed; antianxiety agents may help those who are primarily anxious, and antipsychotics may help those with a psychotic basis to their illness. Another possibility is that all these agents have some sedative properties and act through this common denominator. No one has successfully cross-validated a diagnostic scheme

Table 5.4

The Therapeutic Effects of Doxepin in Anxiety and Depression and in Depression—Comparison of Doxepin with Standard Drug

	Doxepin		
	Superior	Equal	Inferior
Anxiety–depression syndrome			
Placebo	6	0	0
Chlordiazepoxide	0	11	0
Diazepam	1	7	0
Amitriptyline	1	1	0
Amitriptyline–perphenazine	1	4	1
Thioridazine	0	1	0
Depression			
Placebo	2	0	0
Imipramine	0	3	0
Amitriptyline	0	8	0
Amitriptyline–perphenazine	0	1	0

for predicting which drug or combination will be optimal for any patient subgroup with mixed anxiety and depression.

If mixed anxiety-depression should shade into psychotic depression, or if any questions exist as to a basic psychotic process, a phenothiazine-tricyclic antidepressant combination may prove useful. Pure anxiety may respond best to a benzodiazepine antianxiety agent or doxepin, while a hostile depression may improve on antipsychotics. Patients failing to respond to one agent may do well on another.

Anxiety Associated with Physical Illness

Anxiety associated with physical illness has been well studied in double-blind studies, and there is a very large and substantial body of evidence showing beyond a reasonable doubt that benzodiazepine is effective in reducing anxiety in this situation and, furthermore, does so to the same degree that it reduces anxiety as it occurs in anxiety disorders.

Personality Disorders and AA Use

Generally, patients with personality disorders do not improve with drug treatment in a specific or dramatic manner. For these people, psychological intervention is the primary treatment. Although most personality disorders do not respond to psychotropic drugs, some do show excellent improvement. Also, clinical experience indicates that the most useful drugs in some personality disorders are the unexpected ones. Pseudoneurotic schizophrenics may respond to tricyclic antidepressants and not to antipsychotic medication. Emotionally unstable personalities may respond to phenothiazines or lithium and not to minor tranquilizers. Donald Klein, M.D. at the Columbia University College of Physicians and Surgeons has been one of the few to investigate this problem.

Passive Aggressive and Dependent Personality Disorder

Dependent. These patients may respond to antidepressant medication with increased energy, hopefulness and social participation. One reason for this may be that some dependent passive-aggressives are really depressed patients unable to do for themselves because they cannot derive or anticipate pleasure.

Aggressive. Phenothiazines are more effective than AAs, but hard data is lacking.

Schizoptypical Personality Disorders

Treat target symptoms with the appropriate agent. Otherwise, drugs have no effect. Antidepressants may unveil a schizophrenic psychosis in such patients, so use them very carefully. The same considerations apply to paranoid, schizoid, and borderline cases.

Other Disorders

For sexual deviation, we cannot recommend any drug for routine treatment at this time. However, considerable experimental work is being done on hormonal agents (e.g., depo-estrogens (Provera) for certain male sexual deviations and episodic aggression).

There is no drug treatment of pure antisocial personality disorders at this time.

General Remarks

Most neuroses and personality disorders are primarily psychogenic in origin. Occasionally, brief use of antianxiety agents can be helpful for a week or two to take the edge off anxiety, but, in general, the treatment for these conditions is psychological and not pharmacological. There has been little work in this area. We have tried to indicate where some evidence for efficacy of drugs is indicated, but, in general, the use of drugs has not been well investigated. We would stress the importance of psychological therapies for these conditions, and we want to clearly state that medication can be useful only on occasion. There should be no substitute for the primary therapy, which in this case is psychological therapy. These remarks are based on an act of faith. Psychodynamic psychotherapies have not been subject to a great deal of controlled investigation, so it is mainly the authors' clinical opinion that these therapies are useful. Most of the generalizations in this book are about drug efficacy and are backed by overwhelming evidence.

AAs vs. Barbiturates

Effectiveness

The superiority of AA's and barbiturates over a placebo can be consistently shown. However, the superiority of the AA over a barbiturate is not as certain. Nevertheless, many studies suggest that AA's have greater clinical effect.

> **Advantages of AAs Over Barbiturates**
>
> - Less addicting
> - Less drowsiness
> - Less suicide potentiality
> - Less dermatitis
> - Less disinhibiting effect (e.g., excitement in old patients; "goof ball" high in street corner youth)

At doses that produce equal sedation, AAs produce more antianxiety and other therapeutic effects than do the barbiturates. The rationale for this statement is that in clinical trials, sedative side effects are about equal. However, there is generally a slightly superior therapeutic effect with antianxiety agents over the barbiturates. It would be fair to say that there is some evidence that this is true, but there is not a substantial degree of evidence. Differences among the agents are small, such that one is much more struck by their similarities.

Lower class patients often equate feeling sedated with being tranquilized. They welcome this as evidence that the medication is helping. They often experience anxiety through physical distress and identify sickness as the presence of these symptoms. Such patients may consider drug side effects manifestations of sickness. Middle class people, on the other hand, may dislike being sedated and feel that it interferes with mental alertness on the job. Educated patients tend to correctly identify dry mouth or other drug side effects as such, not thinking of them as psychophysiological equivalents of anxiety, and are, therefore, less alarmed by side effects.

AAs vs. Phenothiazines

Antipsychotics are effective against psychotic agitation, whereas AAs are not, and sometimes worsen it.

Although antipsychotics are often used to treat anxiety, we believe this to be a great error. Antipsychotics produce a wide variety of side effects.

- *Atropine*—Blurred vision prevents patients from reading; dry mouth is annoying.
- *Akathisia*—Patients often feel agitated and more upset than they felt before drug therapy.

- *Drowsiness*—Along with akinetic parkinsonism, patients may feel lifeless.
- The danger of *tardive dyskinesia*.

This is the most important side effect of the antipsychotic drugs. Although tardive dyskinesia is long-term and dose-related, and occurs more frequently in patients who have been on antipsychotics for many years, it can occur with low doses and short duration treatment.

These, plus the many other side effects previously enumerated, make phenothiazines too potentially dangerous for neurotic anxiety states. Empirically, some psychoneurotic patients or personality disorders respond dramatically to antipsychotic medication, and not nearly as well to antianxiety medication. While most patients with uncomplicated anxiety should be treated with antianxiety agents for the above reasons, patients who respond poorly may deserve an antipsychotic drug trial. In addition, patients who have had previous psychotic episodes, and those in whom you suspect a psychotic process may warrant a trial on antipsychotic medication.

In comparing antipsychotics with antianxiety agents it is important to remember that AAs also have important side effects. Patients treated with antianxiety agents on a clinical basis for five months developed mild withdrawal symptoms, when the antianxiety agents were discontinued (anxiety, irritability, etc). Although this study does not conclusively prove that withdrawal symptoms can occur on usual doses, it does suggest caution in the use of long-term antianxiety agents. It is possible that these same symptoms were a return of the initial anxiety symptoms, yet the coincidence of the symptoms with cessation of treatment is striking. There is no doubt that antianxiety agents (in amounts only minimally higher than the usual therapeutic dose) do produce barbiturate-type withdrawal symptoms. This attaches an important hazard to the use of antianxiety agents. In addition, although antianxiety agents are less dangerous in the overdose situation than barbiturates, they do have some overdose toxicity. It is particularly important to discontinue AAs since the possibility exists that their long-term use could be similar to a barbiturate-type abuse.

Most authors agree AAs ought to be used only for short-term treatment and are ineffective when given continuously. Up to the present, no placebo-controlled study shows the effectiveness of long-term benzodiazepine treatment for anxiety. This does not mean their effectiveness does not continue over months or years, but only that it has yet to be objectively demonstrated.

CHOOSING AN ANTIANXIETY AGENT

Effectiveness (Table 5.5)

Meprobamate (Equanil; Miltown)

Despite being rated better than placebo in most controlled studies, this drug is continually under attack. Nevertheless, this agent's efficacy is approximately equal to that of barbiturates. Meprobamate is safe for use during pregnancy. After 15 years of use, Ayd reports no deleterious effects in pregnant women.

However, it does have the highest addiction risk of all AA drugs. Withdrawal syndromes occur on as little as four times the usual daily therapeutic dose (3200 mg). Meprobamate also has the highest suicide potential of all the AAs, but less than barbiturates.

Tybamate (Solacen; Tybatran)

This medicine is supposed to be particularly useful in the therapy of treatment-resistant neurotic and anxious medical clinic

Table 5.5
Classification and Dose Range

Drug	Total daily dose (divided into 2–4)
Glycerol derivatives	
Meprobamate (Equanil; Miltown)	800–3200 mg
Tybamate (Solacen; Tybatran)	600–1200 mg
Meprobamate + Benactyzine (Deprol) (400 mg) (1 mg)	1–6 tabs
Benzodiazepines	
Chlordiazepoxide (Librium)	15–300 mg
Diazepam (Valium)	5–60 mg
Oxazepam (Serax)	30–120 mg
Clorazepate dipotassium (Tranxene)	15–60 mg
Flurazepam (Dalmane)	15–30 mg
Lorazepam (Ativan)	1–10 mg
Prazepam (Verstran)	20–60 mg
Diphenylmethane derivatives	
Hydroxyzine (Atarax; Vistaril)	75–400 mg

patients. This controlled finding must be cross-validated, however. Tybamate, rarely (if ever) produces a withdrawal syndrome.

Tybamate, a mild AA which produces few side effects and has antianxiety properties, may be successful with lower class patients, particularly those patients who frequent medical clinics and show multiple somatic complaints and identify drug-induced side effects as symptoms of a disease.

Meprobamate-Benactyzine (Deprol)

Benactyzine is an anticholinergic agent. Deprol is superior to a placebo for treating mild anxiety and depression in outpatients. Although this drug has been shown to be effective in a limited number of double blind studies, Deprol has not been extensively investigated in controlled studies, so we reserve judgment on its efficacy until further information is available.

Benzodiazepines [chlordiazepoxide (Librium); diazepam (Valium); oxazepam (Serax); clorazepate dipotassium (Tranxene); flurazepam (Dalmane); lorazepam (Ativin); prazepam (Verstran)

Most double-blind comparisons find these drugs superior to placebos, but not as many are superior to barbiturates or glycerol derivatives (e.g., meprobamate). These agents have a low suicide potential when taken in overdose. Allegedly, they increase vigor and well being. Benzodiazepines have sedative-hypnotic, anxiolytic, muscle relaxant, and anticonvulsant activities. They are disinhibitory and can restore behavior suppressed by punishment. Fearful avoidance is replaced by freedom to act.

You should use these drugs for preventing delerium tremens and convulsions during acute alcohol withdrawal. They may also be used to control seizure disorders. Diazepam has been used successfully in acute dystonic reactions in doses of 20 to 30 mg by mouth if anticholinergics fail.

For complete comparative studies on the efficacy of antianxiety agents, see Table 5.6.

Chlordiazepoxide (Librium)

This drug is well absorbed orally and blood concentration peaks in several hours. Intramuscular absorption is slow, painful and erratic. The two main metabolites (desmethylchlordiazepoxide

Table 5.6
Comparative Efficacy Studies—Antianxiety Agents

Generic name	Percentage of studies in which		
	Drug was better than placebo	Drug was better than barbiturates	Drug was better than meprobamate
Barbiturates	68% (19)*		—
Meprobamate (Miltown; Equanil)	67% (27)	30% (10)	
Tybamate (Solacen; Tybatran)	94% (16)	nsi†	67% (3)
Chlordiazepoxide (Librium)	96% (28)	43% (7)	20% (5)
Diazepam (Valium)	89% (18)	80% (5)	50% (2)
Oxazepam (Serax)	89% (9)	nsi	nsi

* Numbers in parentheses are total numbers of studies comparing two drugs.

† nsi = not sufficient information available to permit a quantitative comparison.

and demoxepam) are psychopharmacologically active. The half-life varies from 6 to 30 hours among individuals. Because of recently developed pharmacokinetic knowledge, chlordiazepoxide need not be given more than twice daily. This drug may paradoxically increase irritability and hostility ("Librium rage").

Prazepam

Prazepam (Verstran) is a new minor tranquilizer, recently introduced on the market. It has been shown to possess antianxiety properties with minimal sedation similar to the other minor tranquilizers. This should not be surprising, since this drug is also metabolized into the same metabolites as diazepam, and these metabolites possess antianxiety properties. This drug is noted for its long half-life. Blood levels peak at about 6 hours after a single dose. The elimination half-life is about 40–70 hours. Clearly, this drug can be given on once-a-day dosage. Night-time administration can help sleep with some residual effect on daytime anxiety the next day. In terms of therapeutic effects and side effects, it is similar to other drugs in its class.

Clorazepate (Tranxene)

This psychotropic is rapidly transformed to desmethyldiazepam (same as diazepam or prazepam) and has a long half-life, identical to prazepam, since both drugs produce desmethyldiazepam. This drug has been extensively investigated in double-blind, well controlled, randomly assigned studies. It is as effective as the other antianxiety agents.

Diazepam (Valium)

This agent is also rapidly and completely absorbed orally, yet poorly intramuscularly. Peak plasma levels occur in two hours. The half-life of diazepam is 20 to 50 hours. Its major metabolite, desmethyldiazepam, is psychopharmacologically active. Steady-state concentrations are reached after 5 to 10 days because of its long half-life. This must be taken into consideration in the patient who seems to become more lethargic after initial relief from the drug.

Oxazepam (Serax)

This medicine, unlike the previous two, has no active metabolites and a relatively short (4 to 11 hours) half-life. No parenteral form exists. Double-blind studies show that this is as effective an antianxiety agent as Librium and Valium.

Lorazepam (Ativan)

Similar to oxazepam with no active metabolites, it is rapidly inactivated as its three hydroxyl group is directly conjugated to glucuronide. Its elimination half-life is about 12 hours. It has a parenteral form. It has been well studied with a large number of random assignment, double-blind studies, and there is overwhelming evidence that it is an effective antianxiety agent with a high degree of safety. An advantage to both lorazepam and oxazepam is the short half-life, particularly when the medication is taken in response to a specific episode of anxiety. These latter two drugs are inactivated by a rather robust pathway and one less likely to be influenced by liver disease, age, etc., which do slow the metabolism of the other benzodiazepines.

Flurazepam (Dalmane)

This benzodiazepine comes only in oral form. It undergoes Ndealkylation and has a half-life of 50 to 100 hours. It can cause cumulative effects after consecutive use. It is possibly more effective at 30 than at 15 mg. Flurazepam is an effective hypnotic with minimal interference with REM or dreaming sleep. Rarely is it addictive and the danger from overdose is small. It is currently the hypnotic of choice, and does not induce liver microsomal enzymes.

It should be remembered that the differences between flurazepam and the barbiturate or nonbarbiturate hypnotics are often more quantitative than qualitative. There is less liability from overdose than with the barbiturates. There is some potentiality for abuse with flurazepam, but less than with the barbiturates. It should not seem as an innocuous hypnotic, but rather a hypnotic with many of the disadvantages of other hypnotics, only to a quantitatively less degree. There is no evidence that patients do not develop tolerance to flurazepam. It should only be prescribed for short periods of time; there is no evidence that it is effective on a long-term basis.

Use of oxazepam (Serax) and Lorazepam (Ativan) as Hypnotics

Some clinicians use Oxazepam (Serax) or Lorazepam (Ativan) instead of Flurazepam (Dalmane) as a hypnotic because the elimination half-life is much shorter (less than 12 hours versus 50 to 100 hours). Skills are not affected the day after nocturnal drug use. Research is needed to support this clinical practice.

SIDE EFFECTS OF ANTIANXIETY AGENTS

AAs produce remarkably few serious side effects, and blood dyscrasias are rare. The most common side effect is drowsiness. Ataxia sometimes occurs with high doses. Patients can become intoxicated after a few drinks and should be warned to be careful.

Paradoxical rage might be a factor in the rare auto accident that can occur when a patient is treated with antianxiety medication. The benzodiazepine antianxiety agents are less likely to cause barbiturate-type drug dependency than are barbiturates themselves. However, dependency and addiction do occur and can be a problem. For example, chlordiazepoxide given in doses of 300 mg for a month can cause a mild barbiturate-like syndrome. Although successful suicide is unlikely from benzodiazepine-type minor tranquilizers alone, these agents can potentiate other sedatives and may contribute to the total toxic reaction of a patient who takes multiple medications. Meprobamate can be fatal when taken in an overdose, but it is not as lethal as barbiturates.

Drowsiness, ataxia, nystagmus, dysarthria, dizziness, and vertigo are dose-related adverse reactions most likely in elderly patients with low serum albumin. Cutaneous allergies, photosensitivity, nonthrombocytopenic purpura and psychological dependence occur.

References

Phobic Anxiety

Ballenger, J., Sheehan, D., and Jacobson, G.: Antidepressant treatment of severe phobic anxiety. Presented at the Annual Meeting, American Psychiatric Association, Toronto, Canada, May, 1977.

Klein, D. F.: Delineation of two drugs—reserpine anxiety syndromes. Psychopharmacologia 5:397–408, 1964.

Klein, D. F.: Importance of psychiatric diagnosis in the prediction of clinical drug effects. Arch. Gen. Psychiatry 16:118–126, 1967.

Lipsedge, M. S., Hajioff, J., Huggine, P., et al.: The management in severe agoraphobia. Psychopharmacologia 32:67–80, 1973.

Solyom, L., Heseltine, G., McClure, D., et al.: Behavior therapy versus drug therapy in the drug treatment of phobic neurosis. Can. Psychiatr. J. 18:25–31, 1973.

Sheehan, D., Ballenger, J., and Jacobson, G.: The treatment of endogenous anxiety with phobic hysterical and hypochondrical symptoms. Arch. Gen. Psychiatry (in press).

Tyrer, P., Candy, J., and Kelly, D.: A study of the clinical effects of phenelzine and placebo in the treatment of phobic anxiety. Psychopharmacologia 32:237–254, 1973.

Tyrer, P., Candy, J., and Kelly, D.: Phenelzine in phobic anxiety: A controlled trial. Psychol. Med. 3:120–124, 1973.

Zitrin, C. M., Klein, D. F., and Woerner, M. G.: Behavior therapy, supportive psychotherapy, imipramine and pho-

bias. Arch. Gen. Psychiatry 35:307–316, 1972.

General

Cohen, J., Gomez, E., Hoell, N. L., et al.: Diazepam and phenobarbital in the treatment of anxiety: a controlled multicenter study using physician and patient rating scales. Curr. Ther. Res. 20:184–193, 1976.

Covi, L., Lipman, R. S., Derogatis, L. R., et al.: Drugs and group psychotherapy in neurotic depression. Am. J. Psychiatry 131:191–198, 1974.

Covi, L., Lipman, R. S., Pattison, J. H., et al.: Length of treatment with anxiolytic sedatives and response to their sudden withdrawal. Acta Psychiatr. Scand. 49:51–64, 1973.

Davis, J. M., Bartlett, E., and Termini, B. A.: Overdosage of psychotropic drugs. Dis. Nerv. Syst. 29:157–246, 1968.

Dureman, I., and Norrman, B.: Clinical and experimental comparison of diazepam, chlorazepate and placebo. Psychopharmacologia 40:279–284, 1975.

El-yousef, M. K., Janowsky, D. S., Davis, J. M., et al.: Reversal by physostigmine of antiparkinsonian drug toxicity: A controlled study. Am. J. Psychiatry 130:141–145, 1973.

Greenblatt, D. J., and Shader, R. I.: Pharmacotherapy of anxiety with benzodiazepines and β-adrenergic blockers. In *Psychopharmacology: A Generation of Progress* (Lipton, M. A., DiMascio, A., and Killiam, K. F., eds., pp. 1381–1390. New York, Raven Press, 1978.

Greenblatt, D. J., and Shader, R. I.: Prazepam and lorazepam, two new benzodiazepines. New Engl. J. Med. *299:* 1342–1343, 1978.

Greenblatt, D. J., and Shader, R. I.: Prazepam, a precursor of desmethyldiazepam. Lancet 1:720, 1978.

Greenblatt, D. J., Shader, R. I., and Koch-Weser, J.: Serum creatine phosphokinase concentrations after intramuscular chlordiazepoxide and its solvent. J. Clin. Pharmacol. *16:*118–121, 1976.

Greenblatt, D. J., Shader, R. I., MacLeod, S., et al.: Clinical pharmacokinetics of chlordiazepoxide. Clin. Pharmacokinetics 3:381–394, 1978.

Greenblatt, D. J., Shader, R. I., MacLeod, S. M. et al.: Absorption of oral and intramuscular chlordiazepoxide. Eur. J. Clin. Pharmacol. *13:*267–274, 1978.

Greenblatt, D. J., and Shader, R. I.: Benzodiazepines in clinical practice. New York, Raven Press, 1974.

Greenblatt, D. J., and Shader, R. I.: Drug interactions in psychopharmacology. In *Manual of Psychiatric Therapeutics* (Shader, R. I., ed.), pp. 269–279. Boston, Little Brown and Co., 1975.

Goldberg, H. L., and Finnerty, R. J.: A double-blind study of prazepam vs. placebo in single doses in the treatment of anxiety. Comp. Psychiatry *18:*147–156, 1977.

Haider, I.: A comparative trial of RO-4-6270 and amitriptyline in depressive illness, Br. J. Psychiatry *113:*993–998, 1967.

Haizlip, T. M., and Eqing, J. A.: Meprobamate habituation. A controlled clinical study. N. Engl. J. Med. *258:* 1181–1186, 1958.

Hall, R., and Jaffe, J.: Aberrant response to diazepam: A new syndrome. Am. J. Psychiatry *129:*738, 1972.

Hare, H. P.: Comparison of chlordiazepoxide-amitriptyline combination with amitriptyline alone in anxiety-depressive states. J. Clin. Pharmacol. *11:*456–460, 1971.

Hesbacher, P. T., Rickels, K., Gordon, P. E., et al.: Setting, patient and doctor effects on drug response in neurotic patients. I. Differential attrition, dosage deviation and side reaction response to treatment. Psychopharmacologia *18:*180–208, 1970.

Hesbacher, P. T., Rickels, K., Hutchinson, J., et al.: Setting, patient and doctor effects on drug response in neurotic patients. II. Differential improvement. Psychopharmacologia *18:* 209–226, 1970.

Hollister, L. E., and Glazener, F. S.: Withdrawal reactions from meprobamate, alone and combined with promazine: a controlled study. Psychopharmacologia 1:336–341, 1960.

Hollister, L. E., Motzenbecker, F. P., and Degan, R. O.: Withdrawal reactions from chlordiazepoxide ("Librium"), Psychopharmacologia 2:63–68, 1961.

Klotz, U., Avant, G. R., Hoyumpa, A., et al.: The effects of age and liver disease on the disposition and elimination of diazepam in adult man. J. Clin. Invest. *55:*347–359, 1975.

Kraus, J. W., Desmond, P. V., Marshall, J. P., et al.: Effects of aging and liver disease on disposition of lorazepam. Clin. Pharmacol. Ther. *24:*411–419, 1978.

Lader, M. H., Bond, A. J., and James, D. C.: Clinical comparison of anxiolytic drug therapy. Psychol. Med. 4:381–387, 1974.

Lader, M. D., and Wing, L.: Physiological measures, sedative drugs and morbid anxiety. Maudsley Monograph No. 14, p.i. London, Oxford University Press, 1966.

Lipman, P. S., and Covi, L.: Outpatient treatment of neurotic depression: Medication and group psychotherapy. In *Evaluation and Psychological Therapies* (Spitzer, R. G., and Klein, D. F., eds.) Baltimore, Johns Hopkins University Press, 1976.

Lipman, R. S., Hammer, H. M. M., Bernardes, J. F., et al.: Patient report of significant life situation events. Dis. Nerv. Syst. 26:586, 1965.

Lipman, R. S., Covi, L., Derogatis, L. R., et al.: Medication, anxiety reduction and patient report of significant life situation events. Dis. Nerv. Syst. *32:* 240, 1971.

MacLeod, S., Sellers, E., Giles, H., et al.: Interaction of disulfiram with benzodiazepines. Clin. Pharmacol. Ther. *24:* 583–589, 1978.

Magnus, R. V., Dean, B. C., and Curry, S. H.: Clorazepate: double-blind crossover comparison of a single nightly dose with diazepam thrice daily in anxiety. Dis. Nerv. Syst. *38:* 819–821, 1977.

McMillin, W. P.: Oxprenolol in anxiety. Lancet *1:*1193, 1973.

Pevnick, J., Jasenski, D., and Haertzen, C.: Abrupt withdrawal from therapeutically administered diazepam. Arch. Gen. Psychiatry *35:*995–998, 1978.

Ramsey, I., Greer, S., and Bagley, C.: Propranolol in neurotic and thyrotoxic anxiety. Br. J. Psychiatry *122:* 555–560, 1973.

Richards, D. J.: Clinical profile of lorazepam. Dis. Nerv. Syst. *39:*56–66, 1978.

Rickels, K., Hesbacher, P., Vandervort, W., et al.: Tybamate—a perplexing drug. Am. J. Psychiatry *125:*320, 1968.

Rickels, K., and Snow, L.: Meprobamate and phenobarbital sodium in anxious neurotic psychiatric patients and medical clinical outpatients. Psychopharmacologia *5:*339, 1964.

Rickels, K.: Use of antianxiety agents in anxious outpatients. Psychopharmacologia *58:*1–17, 1978.

Rickels, K., Sablosky, H., Silverman, H., et al.: Prazepam in anxiety: a controlled clinical trial. Comp. Psychiatry *18:*239–249, 1977.

Rickels, K., Weise, C. C., Clark, E. L., et al.: Thiothixene and thioridazine in anxiety. Br. J. Psychiatry *125:*79–87, 1974.

Roberts, R. K., Wilkinson, G. R., Branch, R. A., et al.: The effect of age and parenchymal liver disease in the distribution and elimination of chlordiazepoxide (Librium). Gastroenterology *75:*479–485, 1978.

Robin, A., Curry, S. H., and Whelpton, R.: Clinical and biochemical comparison of clorazepate and diazepam. Psychol. Med. *4:*388–392, 1974.

Salzman, C., Kochansky, G. E., Shader, R. I., et al.: Chlordiazepoxide-induced hostility in a small group setting. Arch. Gen. Psychiatry *31:*401–405, 1974.

Schapira, K., McClelland, H., and Newell, D.: A comparison of high and low dose lorazepam with amylobarbitone in patients with anxiety states. Am. J. Psychiatry *134:*25–28, 1977.

Schatzberg, A. F., and Cole, J. O.: Benzodiazepines in depressive disorders. Arch. Gen. Psychiatry *35:*1359–1366, 1978.

Uhlenhuth, E. H., Rickels, K., Fisher, S., et al.: Drug doctor's verbal attitude and clinic setting in the symptomatic response to pharmacotherapy. Psychopharmacologia *9:*392–418, 1966.

Weir, J. H.: Prazepam in the treatment of anxiety. J. Clin. Psychiatry *39:*841, 1978.

Wheatley, D.: Comparative effects of propranolol and chlordiazepoxide in anxiety states. Br. J. Psychiatry *115:* 1411–1412, 1969.

Wheatley, D.: *Psychopharmacology in Family Practice.* London, William Heinemann, Medical Books, Ltd., 1973.

chapter SIX

Medical Emergency: Overdose

A mentally disturbed patient can obtain a prescription for a psychotropic drug from his physician and take the entire bottle in a suicide attempt. Drugs of abuse are also occasionally taken in suicide attempts. Although the initial care of a serious coma secondary to psychotropic drug ingestion may be managed by an internist, you should be familiar with various overdose syndromes, the general principles of management and the specific treatment aspects for each syndrome (see Tables 6.1 and 6.2).

GENERAL ASPECTS OF TREATMENT

Prevention of Further Absorption

- Emesis—hypertonic saline.
- Gastric lavage.
- Cathartics.
- Washing.
- Tourniquet and chilling.

Supportive Treatment

Coma—CNS stimulants controversial.
- Shock—Trendelenburg position, blood or fluids, vasopressors, steroids.
- Respiratory difficulty, hypoxia—clear airway, suction repeatedly, oxygen, mechanical assistance if needed, watch for pulmonary complications.
- Temperature control.
- Renal—catheterize if necessary, watch for adequate output.
- Fluid and electrolyte balance.

Table 6.1
Specific Aspects of Treatment in Drug Overdose*

Drug	Prevention of absorption	Supportive Rx	Specific antidotal treatment
Phenothiazines	Lavage even late (gastric mobility ↓)	Rx hypothermia cautiously, as hyperthermia can occur	Cogentin, Benadryl or caffeine for extrapyramidal Sx Levarterenol for hypotension (epinephrine will aggravate) Hemodialysis useless (protein binding)
Tricyclics		Monitor EKG for arrhythmias, most deaths due to arrhythmias so this is a particularly important aspect of care; seizure can occur	Short-acting barbiturate or prophylactic Valium for convulsions Physostigmine for arrhythmias and coma Forced diuresis useless (renal excretion of free drug is low) Dialysis useless (protein binding)
MAO inhibitors		Observe 24 hr (lag period)	Go ahead and use forced diuresis or dialysis during lag period, if large dose taken Parnate or Nardil excretion enhanced with acidified urine Chlorpromazine for behavioral disturbance (and α-adrenergic blocking effect will also ↓ BP) If BP↑ persists, use phentolamine AVOID: tyramine-containing foods and tricyclics
Lithium			Dialysis is useful

| Meprobamate | As for barbiturates | Monitor urine output if ↓ | Do osmotic diuresis (20% mannitol, 50 ml/hr IV)
Levarterenol for hypotension
If convulsions, use barbiturate very cautiously
Hemodialysis may be necessary |
| Amphetamines | Can lavage late | Isolate, avoid external stimuli | Sedate with chlorpromazine or haloperidol except with DOM (STP) poisoning. Chlorpromazine exacerbates this. Give barbiturate instead
If BP ↑, give rapid-acting α-adrenergic blocker (phentolamine)
Acidify urine (ammonium chloride)
Dialysis helpful |

* ↓ indicates depressed; ↑ indicated accelerated or raised.

Table 6.2
Overdose Symptoms*

A. Stimulants and Hallucinogens

Drug		Symptoms	Mechanism
Amphetamines	CNS	restless, irritable, insomnia DTRs ↑, panic states, suicide, homicide; convulsions, coma; cerebral hemorrhage	—
	Children:	constant twisting and turning, purposeless movements, mumbling, throws body around, screams	
	CV	pallor or flushing, headache, chilliness, arrhythmias, angina, BP ↑ or ↓, shock	
	Pupils	mydriasis	
	Temp	↑	
	GI	dry mouth, metallic taste, anorexia, nausea, vomiting, diarrhea, abdominal cramps	
	LD:	few deaths, wide safety margin (500 mg survived; 120 mg fatal)	
Atropine drugs	CNS	↑ excited, confused, acute organic psychosis, visual hallucinations, coma	
	Resp	↓ when severe	
	CV	hot, dry red skin, P ↑, BP ↑, when severe → shock	
	Pupils	mydriasis, nonreactive	
	Temp	↑	
	GI	dry mouth, nausea, vomiting	

B. Antipsychotic Drugs

Phenothiazines		
CNS	↓ drowsy → coma, DTRs ↓	Extrapyramidal tract stimulation
CV	BP ↓, P ↑ rarely, arrhythmias	
Pupils	miosis	
Temp	↓	
CNS with piperazines: restless, tremor, twitching, spasm, rigid, convulsions		
Dosage: death is rare even with large doses		

C. Antidepressants

Tricyclics		
CNS	↓ may have delirium, agitation, before onset of coma, DTRs ↑, convulsions	Hypotension; toxic to myocardium (aggravated by ↑ workload due to tachycardia)
Resp	↓	
CV	BP ↑ or ↓, P ↑ shock may occur atrial fibrillation ventricular flutter } especially in children AV block	
Pupils	mydriasis	
Temp	↑	
Late death	after several days, cardiac arrest alternating agitation and drowsiness	
Children:		
Dose:	LD is 10–30 × daily dosage	

Table 6.2—continued

Drug	Symptoms	Mechanism
	C. Antidepressants	
MAO inhibitors	Lag period—watch	
	CNS motor uneasiness, agitation, violent motor activity (with moaning, grimacing), hallucinations, convulsions, coma	
	Resp ↑	
	CV BP ↑ or ↓, P ↑	
	Pupils mydriasis	
	Temp ↑ sweating	
	Doses: 5000 mg fatal; 375 mg fatal; 170 mg fatal, 350 mg survived	
	D. Antimanics	
Lithium	CNS muscles hypertonic, tremors, DTRs ↑, grunts, convulsions, transitory neurologic asymmetries simulating cerebral hemorrhage, coma	
	Resp complications: atelectasis, pneumonia	
	Dose: very narrow margin of safety	

E. Antianxiety Agents

Benzodiazepines	CNS	drowsy, lethargic, coma is rare
	Resp	slightly ↓
	CV	BP, P slightly ↓
	No deaths:	up to 2¼ g Librium survived
Meprobamate	CNS	drowsy, coma, occasional paradoxical excitement, seizures
	Resp	→
	CV	BP ↓
	Temp	→
	Complications: atelectasis, pulmonary edema
	Dose:	12 g fatal; 40 g survived

* ↓ indicates depressed; ↑ indicates accelerated or raised. NL = nonlethal dose.

- Bed care—turn frequently, keep bed dry.
- Prophylaxis for phlebothrombosis.
- Control of convulsions—use short-acting barbiturate.

Specific Antidotal Treatments

- Biochemical competition for site.
- Antagonistic action.
- Promotion of excretion.

Reference

Shader, R. I. (ed.): *Manual of Psychiatric Therapies: Practical Psychopharmacology and Psychiatry.* Boston, Little, Brown, 1975.

Index

75091